Applied
equine nutrition
and training

Equine NUtrition and TRAining COnference
(ENUTRACO) 2011

edited by: Arno Lindner

Arbeitsgruppe Pferd

Wageningen Academic
P u b l i s h e r s

Photos cover:
Sabine Heueveldop
Sarah Ralston
Manfred Coenen
Marco Polettini

ISBN: 978-90-8686-183-5
e-ISBN: 978-90-8686-740-0
DOI: 10.3920/978-90-8686-740-0

First published, 2011

© **Wageningen Academic Publishers**
The Netherlands, 2011

Wageningen Academic Publishers
P.O. Box 220
6700 AE Wageningen
the Netherlands
www.WageningenAcademic.com
copyright@WageningenAcademic.com

Applied equine nutrition and training

Table of contents

Expanded abstracts

Editorial

We made it: the 4th Equine Nutrition and Training Conference is up and running! Proof is this book. My congratulations and gratitude to all those involved, with special mention of our partners from Vetoquinol/ Equistro as well as Lohmann Animal Health/Lonza! I thoroughly enjoyed organising and even more so the hosting of this meeting and wish to be able to hold another one in 2013! With a 'little help of my friends' this should be made possible!

The aim of the articles in this book is to present and discuss the latest scientific findings on nutrition and training of horses (News) and to provide practical advice to the readers. It would be too much of a challenge to present everything on nutrition and training in one conference, and therefore, the selection of the references in the articles on News depends on the authors' choices. Combined with the discussions during the conference these presentations should allow the participants a good insight into each one of the selected subjects (please also join us in 2013!). The articles on practical advice are very informative and functional, including in some cases that (practical) information is lacking or statistically insignificant but practically very relevant.

Finally, the expanded abstracts on actual and focused research aspects are of excellent additional value to the section on nutrition and training of horses in the book. Thank you very much to these authors for submitting the work in the definite format, going through the reviewing process to present at the conference and the willingness to publish the work in this book!

I wish that all those reading the articles find lots of interesting and useful information! Please send me an e-mail (arnolindner@t-online.de) and comment on what you would be interested in! Maybe we can consider it for 2013!

Wish you health and fun!
Arno

Articles

Practical news on equine nutrition for the breeder published in scientific literature between 2009-2011

Géraldine Blanchard
Animal Nutrition Expertise SARL, 33, Av. de l'île de France, 92160 Antony, France; gb@vet-nutrition.com

After wide considerations of the foal's growth in the early 2000's, recent publications concerning breeding have focused on a variety of topics that we'll consider in the chronology of breeding. Starting with mares and stallions, the potential interactions of nutrition and fertility can be examined considering the athlete or racing career on one hand, and the body condition and metabolism on the other hand. The relationship between nutrition and the oestrus cycle and fertility, especially in the maiden mare is an interesting and practical approach. Then the interaction between the mare's nutrition and the foal's metabolism has been studied. The third topic is on the selenium supplementation of the stallion or the mare, and the consequences on the foal's health. Clinical nutrition will close this review.

Fertility

Stallions and mares may have two parallel careers, one as a genitor, and one as an athlete, that could affect each other. To evaluate the effects of racing on fertility in Standardbred and Finnhorse, the career of stallions and mares were followed in not less than 75,000 mares (Sairannen *et al.*, 2011). In these two breeds the genetic correlation between best racing record and fertility was weak or negligible, at least in this study. It showed also that the stallion fertility did not suffer from racing during the mating year. But for mares, the situation may be much more diverse. The most negative situation was for mares, racing after the first mating or more than 10 times during the mating year, as it diminished the foaling outcome. However, racing only before the first mating or 1 to 5 times during the mating year had positive effects on mare fertility. Finally, the mares with the best career racing records had the highest foaling rates. The authors emphasized that this feature was probably due to preferential treatment (nutrition, environment, close follow up of fertility...). If this explanation is confirmed, that would signify that the best care may compensate a demanding situation in the mares with the best potential. But to estimate the variable with the highest impact, more data will be necessary including studies of other breeds or race types than Finnhorse and Standardbred.

Metabolism/body condition

Mares can suffer from being overweight, with consequences on their glucose and insulin metabolism and the risk for metabolic syndrome. Standardbred maiden mares are considered stressed and in poor physical condition at the end of their racing careers, due to incorrect management (Vecchi *et al.*, 2010). The estimation of body condition score (BCS) and fat thickness by ultrasound method provided similar results. In Standardbred maiden mares of various ages, both BCS and fat thickness were significantly and reciprocally correlated to the time of first seasonal ovulation. In other terms, in stressed maiden mares with low condition score, a flushing or nutrition plane started about 3 weeks before the breeding season may stimulate ovarian activity (Vecchi *et al.*, 2010). These data, together with data on pony mares (Dugdale *et al.*, 2010) which confirm the huge potential appetite of mares, should encourage feeding mares properly but not excessively all year long, adapting the diet to maintain a proper body condition.

Even if in breeding areas, the use of pasture is maximized, concentrate feeding is usually considered beneficial to mares (Karren *et al.*, 2010), and often necessary, at least to provide minerals, trace-elements and vitamins lacking in forage. Beside forage, supplement feeds may be provided. But the mare's tolerance for starch might differ with pregnancy.

Starch-rich feed supplements appear to be better tolerated by pregnant than non-pregnant mares (George *et al.*, 2011). This applies for mares of optimal body condition. The fact that pregnancy enhances glycemic and insulinemic effects of starch-rich concentrate may be explained by the increased requirements, including energy and glucose requirements associated with pregnancy in all mammal females. But if the mare receives a high level of starch-rich feeds, the effects on the mare and the foal's metabolism have to be considered. The number of meals may also have an impact. This has been partly answered in foals from mares receiving two-thirds of their diet from low or high starch feed in late gestation. The offspring showed a significant difference in blood glucose 80 days after birth, but always within normal range, and a trend in insulin sensitivity at 160 days (George *et al.*, 2009). More data on the long-term consequences of this trend are required to understand the importance of the findings.

Selenium/anti-oxidant

Anti-oxidant supplementation of stallions may have an impact on the semen characteristics. In the case of a basic diet, the addition of organic selenium, vitamin E and zinc in stallions lead to an improvement of various sperm characteristics: velocity, straightness, viability, progressive motility, accompanied by an increase of the total seminal plasma antioxidant level and a decrease of abnormal sperm morphology (Contri *et al.*, 2011). These positive consequences may appear quite late, only after 30 to 60 days of supplementation. However, to prevent any negative over supplementation, at first, the composition of the entire diet of the stallion must be considered before adding selenium and other anti-oxidants.

Mares and foals benefit from receiving a grain mix fed providing 100% and furthermore 120% of the selenium amount recommended by the NRC (National Research Council, USA). The mare's colostrum and the foal's plasma and muscle show a higher selenium concentration with supplementation of the mare during the 110 days preceding parturition (Karren *et al.*, 2010). But selenium supplementation had no effect on foaling variables and on the composition of colostrum (Thorson *et al.*, 2010). Furthermore, mares on pasture with no feed supplementation showed the greatest IG concentration in colostrum. However, this must be interpreted with caution, considering the composition of the feed. The supplementation with anti-oxidants can not be limited to the concentration of the trace-element in body fluids (Calamari *et al.*, 2010; Muirhead *et al.*, 2010). Finally, in mares as in stallions, prior to adding supplemental selenium, concentrate feed must be evaluated in order to consider the total amount of nutrients.

Clinical nutrition

Two reviews are of interest, one for pregnant and lactating pony mares, especially overweight ones, at risk of hyperlipemia while losing appetite (McKenzie, 2011), and one for feeding management of the sick foal (McKenzie and Geor, 2009).

Due to the lack of information on the young foal requirements especially when sick, foals' nutrition is a challenge for breeders, practitioners and even nutritionists. A review of the feeding management of the sick foal is available (McKenzie and Geor, 2009), including enteral nutrition, enteral support and how to provide it, from the neonate to weaning, parenteral nutrition including short term caloric supplementation, formulation, administration and monitoring of parenteral nutrition and insulin therapy when required. As an example, the foals energy requirement, including basal metabolism and growth, is about 150 kcal/kg body weight/day in neonates, and decreases progressively to 80 to 100 kcal/kg body weight/day by 1 to 2 months of age. Due to the difference between mare's (about 64%, 22% and 13% of dry matter as sugar, protein, and fat, respectively) and cow milk (about 38%, 26% and 30% of dry matter as sugar, protein, and fat, respectively), the feeding of the foal has to be specific and requires the endogenous production of insulin by the pancreatic b-cells. This function is related to endocrine function, itself linked to the nutrient composition of the milk. The foal's nutrition characteristics are still not fully known, and the management of the sick foal must include at least what is already understood, even if it would require further work.

References

Calamari L, Abeni F, Bertin G (2010) Metabolic and hematological profiles in mature horses supplemented with different selenium sources and doses. J Anim Sci 88:650-659.

Contri A, De Amicis I, Molinari A, Faustini M, Gramenzi A, Robbe D, Carluccio A (2011) Effect of dietary antioxidant supplementation on fresh semen quality in stallion. Theriogenology 75:1319-1326.

Dugdale AH, Curtis GC, Cripps PJ, Harris PA, Argo CM (2010) Effects of season and body condition on appetite, body mass and body composition in *ad libitum* fed pony mares. Vet J (in press).

George LA, Staniar WB, Treiber KH, Harris PA, Geor RJ (2009) Insulin sensitivity and glucose dynamics during pre-weaning foal development and in response to maternal diet composition. Domest Anim Endocrinol 37.23-29.

George LA, Staniar WB, Cubitt TA, Treiber KH, Harris PA, Geor RJ (2011) Evaluation of the effects of pregnancy on insulin sensitivity, insulin secretion, and glucose dynamics in Thoroughbred mares. Am J Vet Res 72:666-674.

Karren BJ, Thorson JF, Cavinder CA, Hammer CJ, Coverdale JA (2010) Effect of selenium supplementation and plane of nutrition on mares and their foals: selenium concentrations and glutathione peroxidase. J Anim Sci 88:991-997.

McKenzie HC (2011) Equine hyperlipemias. Vet Clin North Am Eq Pract 27:59-72.

McKenzie HC, Geor RJ (2009) Feeding management of sick neonatal foals. Vet Clin North Am Eq Pract 25:109-119.

Muirhead TL, Wichtel JJ, Stryhn H, McClure JT (2010) The selenium and vitamin E status of horses in Prince Edward Island. Can Vet J 51:979-985.

Sairanen J, Katila T, Virtala AM, Ojala M (2011) Effects of racing on equine fertility. Anim Reprod Sci 124:73-84.

Thorson JF, Karren BJ, Bauer ML, Cavinder CA, Coverdale JA, Hammer CJ (2010) Effect of selenium supplementation and plane of nutrition on mares and their foals: foaling data. J Anim Sci 88:982-990.

Vecchi I, Sabbioni A, Bigliardi E, Morini G, Ferrari L, Di Ciommo F, Superchi P, Parmigiani F (2010) Relationship between body fat and body condition score and their effects on estrous cycles of the Standardbred maiden mare. Vet Res Commun 34 Suppl 1:S41-S45.

The rider's interaction with the horse

Hilary M. Clayton
Mary Anne McPhail Chair in Equine Sports Medicine, Professor of Large
Animal Clinical Sciences, College of Veterinary Medicine, Michigan State
University, East Lansing, MI 48824, USA; claytonh@cvm.msu.edu

The rider communicates with the horse on several levels, some of which can be measured mechanically. To date, most of these studies have involved using electronic pressure mats to measure pressure distribution on the horse's back and strain gauge transducers to measure tension in the reins. The results are providing information that can be used to develop an understanding of the mechanics of the rider's interaction with the horse.

The horse's thoracolumbar spine behaves as a beam suspended at each end by the forelimbs acting through the thoracic sling muscles, primarily *serratus ventralis*, and by the hind limbs acting through the pelvic girdle. The middle part of the beam tends to sag due to extension of the intervertebral joints under the influence of gravity. The amount of intervertebral extension is controlled by passive (ligamentous) and active (muscular) tension. When a weight is added to the horse's back, it causes the intervertebral joints to extend further bringing the dorsal spinous processes and the articular facets into closer approximation with the consequent risks of impinging spinous processes and facet arthritis. Thus, trainers should teach the horse to maintain roundness of the back under the rider's weight to reduce the risk of spinal injury and associated back pain. The head and neck act as a beam that extends out in front of the body mass and stabilized at its base. During locomotion the base of the neck moves with the horse's shoulders but the upper neck oscillates under the effects of gravity and inertia. These movements affect the horse's contact with the bit.

Saddle pressure measurement

The force of the saddle acting on the horse's back is measured using an electronic pressure mat inserted between the saddle and the horse's back. In the McPhail Equine Performance Center, we use the Pliance mat (Novel Electronics Inc., St. Paul, MN, USA) which has been shown to provide accurate and reliable data (De Cocq *et al.*, 2009), which is not the case for all types of pressure mats. The Pliance mat has 256 sensors distributed in two rectangular mats that are placed on the left and right sides of the horse's back. They are separated across the dorsal midline to avoid the problem of having sensors activated by the sides of the mat being pulled downwards which might suggest that the saddle is impinging on the dorsal spinous processes when this is not the case. Forces registered by the sensors are transmitted to a laptop computer using Bluetooth technology. Since there are no wires connecting the mat to the computer, the horse and rider can move freely while pressures are being measured. The Pliance software calculates the total force on the horse's back by adding the forces on all the individual sensors and provides a colour-coded map of the pressure distribution. A drawback in the use of the saddle mat is that the sensors only register forces that are applied perpendicular to their surface. Shear forces are not measured but can contribute significantly to damage to the skin.

The pressure pattern on the horse's back is displayed in color on the computer screen with black representing the lowest pressure and increasing through blue, cyan, green, yellow, red and pink, which represents the highest pressure. Three types of graphs display the pressure patterns (Figure 1). Numerical analyses are facilitated by subdivision of the total area of the mat transversely (left and right halves) or longitudinally (front, middle, rear sections). The mat provides dynamic data during ridden exercise with real time display of the changing pressure patterns on the computer screen. However, this also complicates the process of analysis since each stride is represented by numerous data points for each sensor. One of the challenges for researchers is to develop analytical procedures that take account of both the spatial and temporal distribution of the forces and pressures on the horse's back.

Saddle fit can be evaluated qualitatively by an experienced saddle fitter under static conditions. The electronic pressure mat has the advantages of measuring the pressure not only at rest but also during locomotion at different gaits.

A well-fitting saddle shows pressure distributed evenly over long, wide panels. When the tree is either too wide or too narrow, the

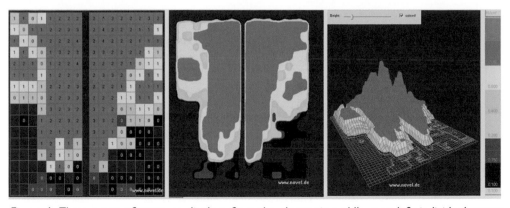

Figure 1. Three types of pressure displays from the electronic saddle mat: left: individual sensor readout; middle: 2D contour pattern; right: 3D contours. All three displays are colour-coded as shown by the key on the right.

pressure is concentrated over a smaller area. With a narrow tree, a common problem is bridging, in which pressure is concentrated in the front and back of the panels with the middle part being unweighted (Harman, 1997) and particularly high pressure at the back of the saddle (Meschan et al., 2006). If the tree is too wide, pressure increases in the middle part of the panels (Meschan et al., 2006). Focal pressure concentrations most often occur over the shoulders when the tree is too narrow, beneath the stirrup bars if the bars are too tight, and along the edge of the panels if their slope does not match the slope of the horse's back (Figure 2).

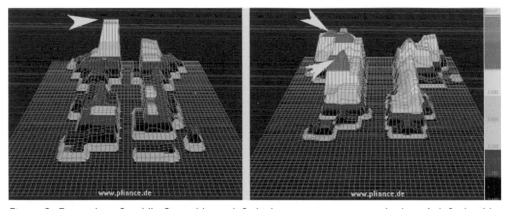

Figure 2. Examples of saddle fit problems: left: high pressure area over the horse's left shoulder (white arrowhead); right: high pressure areas over the left shoulder and beneath the left stirrup bar (white arrowheads).

The use of a pad between the saddle and the horse's back may even out the pressure in saddles that are basically the correct size and shape. Sheepskin has performed particularly well in my own studies (Figure 3) and Kotschwar *et al.* (2010a) have shown a similar beneficial effect with reindeer fur pads in saddles that are basically a good fit for the horse. In poorly fitting saddles, however, different types of pads were beneficial at different gaits. For example, when the saddle tree was too wide, foam and gel pads were most effective at walk whereas gel and reindeer fur were more effective at trot (Kotschwar *et al.*, 2010b).

The tree of the saddle distributes the weight of saddle and rider over a large area of the horse's back. This is in contrast to riding with a treeless saddle or riding bareback when the forces are concentrated beneath the rider's ischial tuberosities.

One of the essentials of riding is to mount the horse. During mounting, the highest total force occurs as the rider's leg swings over the horse's back and this force was significantly higher when the rider mounts from the ground compared with using a mounting block. More importantly, the pressure distribution during mounting is highly asymmetrical on the left and right sides. Pressure is highest on the right side of the withers, which stabilizes the saddle as the rider puts weight on the left stirrup. The left side of the withers is unweighted but there is an area of high pressure on the horse's left shoulder. The horse

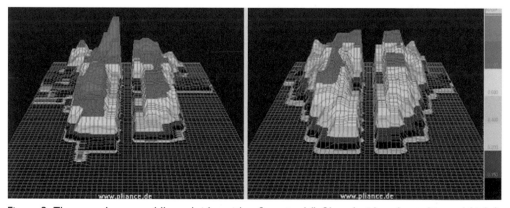

Figure 3. The same horse, saddle and rider with a foam pad (left) and with a sheepskin pad (right). Note the more even pressure distribution with the sheepskin pad compared with the areas of high pressure at the shoulder and under the bars, especially on the left side with foam pad.

braces himself to withstand this asymmetric loading pattern, and it is easy to speculate that this could be associated with uneven muscle development in the left and right shoulders, which is frequently identified by veterinarians and saddle fitters. It is recommended that riders should mount without using the stirrup by either getting a leg up or by using a high enough platform to step onto the horse without using the stirrup. If there is no option to mounting using the stirrup, a mounting block should be used and the rider should switch between mounting from the left and right sides. This will be a positive step toward making the horse straight and symmetrical.

There are large differences between riders in how much force they apply to the horse's back when they land in the saddle; a soft landing is definitely preferable from the horse's standpoint. Some riders have a habit of stepping down forcefully into the right stirrup to center the saddle which has been pulled to the left side during mounting. This is associated with high forces on the horse's back.

Rein tension measurements

Rein tension is easily measured using strain gauges inserted into the rein (Clayton *et al.*, 2005). These sensors measure rein tension dynamically but are unable to distinguish whether the tension originates in the rider pulling on the rein or the horse pushing against the bit. A study using side reins in horses trotting in a straight line showed that there are two peaks in rein tension during each stride of trot and these occur during the diagonal stance phases. The tension increases are caused by the fact that the head and neck nod downwards under the influence of gravity and inertia during the stance phases. Minimal tension, maximal tension and mean tension are all useful measurements that provide different types of information about the rein contact. All three tension variables increase as the reins are shortened. Minimal tension increases and maximal tension decreases with elasticity of the rein (Figure 4) (Clayton *et al.*, 2011).

When a rider is present, riding style has a large effect on tension recordings. For example, dressage training requires the horse to seek contact with the bit resulting in higher rein tension values than for horses trained, for example, in Western riding in which the reins hang loosely. These stylistic differences make it difficult to compare results

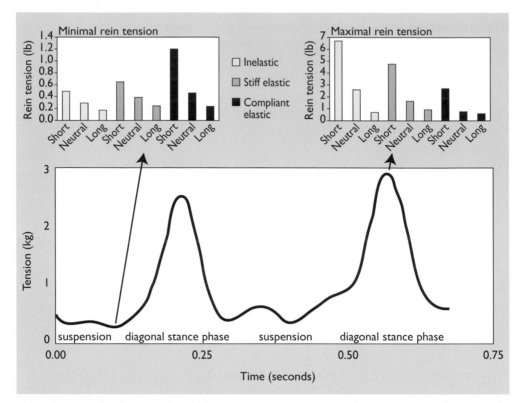

Figure 4. Example of rein tension during one stride at trot using inelastic side reins adjusted to the length of the horse's neck when the horse was standing in a relaxed position. The graph shows the undulating pattern of the tension. The bar charts above show the minimal and maximal rein tensions for an inelastic rein (light bars), a stiff elastic rein (medium bars) and a compliant elastic rein (dark bars). Each rein was adjusted to the neutral length (equal to neck length when standing in a relaxed position), a short length (10 cm shorter than neutral) and a long length (10 cm longer than neutral).

across different studies. My own studies using horses trained in dressage have shown two distinct tension peaks during each stride of trot, whereas at canter there are three peaks per stride, one large peak flanked by two smaller peaks that represent the three-beat rhythm of the canter. In some riders the left and right reins show very similar magnitude and timing of the rein tension oscillations, other riders have differences in the magnitude of left and right rein tensions or in the timing of the tension changes on the left and right sides.

Bitting studies

Radiographic and fluoroscopic studies (Clayton and Lee, 1984; Manfredi *et al.*, 2005) have investigated the position and action of different bits in the horse's mouth. The more recent series of studies used the bits shown in Figure 5. The corresponding lateral radiographs are shown in Figure 6.

The mouthpiece of the single jointed snaffle hangs downwards on the tongue with the joint protruding toward the roof of the mouth where it can put pressure on the underlying bone of the hard palate. When tension is applied to the reins, the mouthpiece becomes more deeply embedded in the tongue, so it moves away from the palate.

The KK Ultra is a double-jointed bit with a short oval-shaped middle piece. Unlike a single jointed snaffle, it has a smooth surface facing toward the palate. Rein tension moves the entire mouthpiece of this bit away from the palate by compressing the tongue. The relatively large separation of the metal from the palate, combined with the

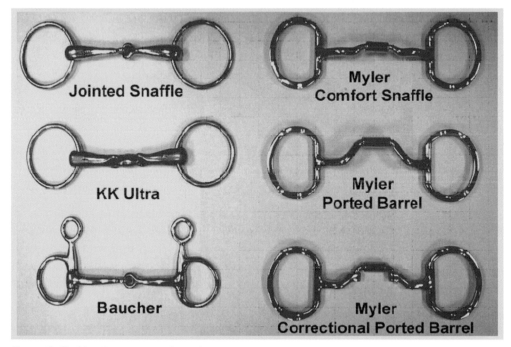

Figure 5. Six bits that were evaluated.

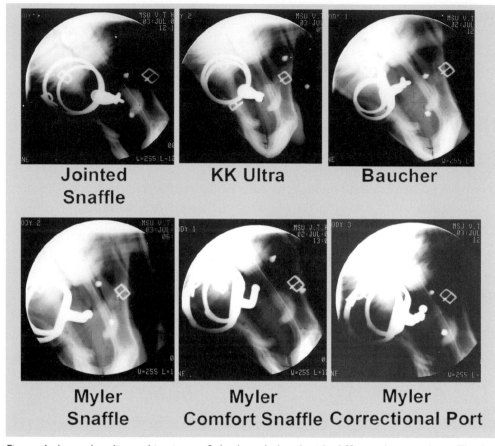

Figure 6. Lateral radiographic views of the horse's head with different bits in place. The bits correspond to those shown in Figure 5.

smoothness of the surface of the central link, may explain why many horses perform well in this bit.

The Baucher bit has an upper ring for attachment of the cheek pieces and a lower ring for attachment of the reins, which gives the bit a more stable position in the horse's mouth when tension is applied to the reins. The joint lies close to the palate and, since the mouthpiece has relatively little mobility, it is difficult for the horse to move this bit inside the oral cavity. Consequently, this may be an uncomfortable bit for some horses.

The two arms of a Myler bit meet within a central barrel that allows a swiveling motion but does not permit any nutcracker action. All three Myler mouthpieces were positioned relatively high on the tongue and the barrel prevents any squeezing action on the tongue. The horse may be able to use his tongue to push against the mouthpiece, giving him a degree of control over the position of the bit and the areas affected by pressure.

Fluoroscopic analysis of the horses' behaviours with the different bits with loose reins and with tension applied to the reins showed a range of intra-oral behaviours that included opening the mouth, retracting the tongue beneath the bit, bulging the middle part of the dorsum of the tongue over the bit and using the tongue to raise the bit between the premolar teeth (Manfredi *et al.*, 2010). Behaviours other than holding the bit quietly in the mouth or chewing gently increased when tension was applied to the reins. The behaviours shown were consistent within each individual horse when wearing different bits but were not specific for the type of bit.

References

Clayton HM, Lee RL (1984) A fluoroscopic study of the position and action of the jointed snaffle bit in the horse's mouth. J Eq Vet Sci 4:193-196.

Clayton HM, Singleton WH, Lanovaz JL, Cloud GL (2005) Strain gauge measurement of rein tension during riding: A pilot study. Eq Comp Exerc Physiol 2:203-205.

De Cocq P, Clayton HM, Terada K, Muller M, van Leeuwen J (2009) Usability of normal force distribution measurements to evaluate asymmetrical loading of the back of the horse and different rider positions on a standing horse. Vet J 181:266-273.

Geutens CA, Clayton HM, Kaiser LJ (2008) Forces and pressures beneath the saddle during mounting from the ground and from a raised mounting block. Vet J 175:332-337.

Harman J (1997) Measurement of the pressures exerted by saddles on the horse's back using a computerized pressure measuring device. Pferdeheilkunde 13:129-134.

Kotschwar AB, Baltacis A, Peham C (2010a) The effects of different saddle pads on forces and pressure distribution beneath a fitting saddle. Eq Vet J 42:114-118.

Kotschwar AB, Baltacis A, Peham C (2010b) The influence of different saddle pads on force and pressure changes beneath saddles with excessively wide trees. Vet J 184:322-325.

Manfredi JM, Rosenstein D, Lanovaz JL, Nauwelaerts S, Clayton HM (2010) Flouroscopic study of oral behaviours in response to the presence of a bit and the effects of rein tension. Comp Exerc Physiol 64:143-148.

Manfredi J, Clayton HM, Rosenstein D (2005) Radiographic study of bit position within the horse's oral cavity. Eq Comp Exerc Physiol 2:195-201.

Meschan E, Peham C, Schobesberger H, Licka T (2007) The influence of the width of the saddle tree on the forces and the pressure distribution under the saddle. Vet J 173: 578-584.

Training techniques to reduce the risk of back injury

Hilary M. Clayton
Mary Anne McPhail Chair in Equine Sports Medicine, Professor of Large Animal Clinical Sciences, College of Veterinary Medicine, Michigan State University, East Lansing, MI 48824, USA; claytonh@cvm.msu.edu

The horse's back plays a crucial role in locomotion and performance. Injuries and diseases of the back occur frequently and are most commonly manifest as a reduction in performance rather than overt lameness, which may pose a diagnostic dilemma. One of our areas of research focus in the McPhail Center is the diagnosis, treatment and prevention of back pain in horses.

Vertebral anatomy

Horses usually have 18 thoracic vertebrae, 6 lumbar vertebrae and 5 fused sacral vertebrae, though the number may vary and anomalies may be found especially in the transitional zones. Conformational differences in the length of the horse's back are a result of differences in either the number of vertebrae or the length of the bodies of the individual vertebrae. Long-backed horses usually have longer vertebral bodies than short-backed horses. This affects the amount of deviation resulting from a change in angle at the joint(s); longer vertebrae deviate further than shorter vertebrae. This means that a long-backed horse shows more lateral displacement for the same angular change at the joints than a short-backed horse. In practical terms, a long-backed horse requires less change in angle at the intervertebral joints than a short-backed horse to achieve the same amount of displacement of the shoulders relative to the haunches when performing a shoulders-in or of the haunches when performing a travers or renvers. It is not unusual for the last lumbar vertebra to be fused to the sacrum so that there are, effectively, only five lumbar vertebrae.

Muscles

The 'bow and string' theory indicates that the horse's spine acts like a bow that can be flexed by contraction of the muscles below the spine. These include the abdominal muscles and the sublumbar muscles. The abdominal muscles (transverse, internal oblique, external oblique, *rectus abdominis*) surround the horse's belly in layers. Their actions include supporting and protecting the internal organs, pressurizing the abdominal cavity and moving the back. The transverse muscle is particularly important for stabilizing the spine in preparation for and during movement. It acts in concert with the epaxial muscles, specifically the *multifidi*. The oblique abdominal muscles assist in stabilizing, flexing and bending the back. The *rectus abdominis* muscle also plays a role in flexing the back.

The sublumbar muscles (*iliopsoas, psoas minor*) are inside the horse's abdomen running from the underside of the vertebrae in the area behind the saddle to the front of the horse's pelvis and femur. Their actions are to pull the front of the pelvis forward (tilt the pelvis) and pull the femur forward (flex the hip). These actions engage the hind limb under the horse's body.

The back muscles lie on either side of the dorsal spinous processes (Figure 1). They can be divided functionally into two groups: the long back muscles and the short back muscles. The long back muscles (*longissimus, iliocostalis*) have long fibers spanning the entire length of the back. When these muscles contract simultaneously on the left and right sides they hollow the back. When they contract unilaterally, they assist in bending the back sideways. The long back muscles have a global effect along the length of the back but they are not able to isolate their effect to a specific spinal segment. The short back muscles (m. *multifidi*) are underneath the long back muscles and lie adjacent to the vertebral spine (Figure 1). The short back muscles act on a single intervertebral joint or up to four adjacent joints, so they have a much more localized effect on a specific joint than the long back muscles. During locomotion, the short back muscles act together with the transverse abdominal muscle to stabilize the horse's back, especially during highly collected movements and in movements such as flying changes in which the back must provide stability to transmit propulsive forces from the hind limbs. An important point

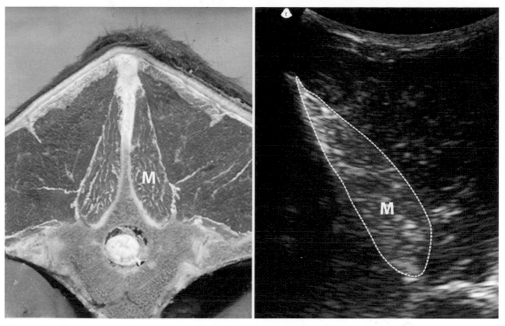

Figure 1. Cross-sectional anatomy of the epaxial muscles. Right: anatomical specimen; left: ultrasonographic image. Note the white fibrous tissue visible within the multifidi in the anatomical view that distinguishes the multifidi from the adjacent longissimus muscle in the ultrasonographic scan. M: multifidus muscle.

to note is that the stabilizing muscles (transverse abdominal muscle and the short back muscles) should be preactivated in anticipation of movement.

Horses and their riders need to develop strength and control of their core musculature both to perform effectively and to protect against developing back pain.

Back mechanics

The thoracolumbar spine is supported by the forelimbs at the withers and by the hind limbs at the croup. Between these supports, the back tends to sag due to the weight of the internal organs. When a rider sits on the horse's back, the extra weight causes the back to extend even more. As the back hollows, the intervertebral joints extend which brings the dorsal spinous processes and articular facets into closer approximation with the consequent risk of bony impingement.

The weight of the rider should be appropriate to the size of the horse to avoid over-extension of the intervertebral joints. As a general recommendation, the rider should not exceed 20% of the horse's weight.

During training, the horse is taught to use the core muscles to maintain flexion of the intervertebral joints even under the rider's weight. This implies using the abdominal and sublumbar muscles to overcome the natural tendency of the back to extend. At the same time, the transverse abdominal muscle and the short back muscles stabilize the intervertebral joints in that rounded position. The horse needs to learn when and how to activate and use these muscles to round the back and then must strengthen the muscles so that the roundness can be maintained throughout the training session.

Lateral bending is achieved by differential contraction of the left and right long back muscles and oblique abdominal muscles. When a horse bends correctly around a turn or circle, the limbs should remain vertical while the intervertebral joints bend to match the curvature of the turn. The smaller the radius of the turn, the more bending is required and the harder the muscles must work to create that bend. This supports the practice of working on large circles and then decreasing the diameter as the bending muscles become stronger. The natural way for a horse to turn is to lean his body to the inside while swinging the neck to the outside of the circle line as a counterbalance. A young horse under saddle falls onto the inside shoulder rather than lifting the shoulder and bending to the inside. Again, the horse must learn to activate the appropriate muscles and coordinate their action with other stabilizing muscles.

Back pathology

The thoracolumbar spine is the site of numerous pathological lesions (Haussler *et al.*, 1999; Stubbs et al, 2010). Many of these injuries are a consequence of the effects of the rider's weight causing extension of the horse's back, which predisposes to impingement of the dorsal spinous processes (kissing spines) and facet joint arthritis. Kissing spines vary in their clinical presentation; some cases are asymptomatic, others are exquisitely painful. Affected horses may resent being saddled, refuse to stand to be mounted, appear cold-backed or show bad behavior, such as bucking or rearing, when ridden. Facet arthritis causes pain and/or stiffness during movement, often resulting in limited range of motion at the affected level on the affected side. However, the majority of horses with back pain show only a reduction in performance (Denoix, 1998; Haussler, 1999)

In people who have unilateral low back pain, the *multifidi* are inhibited and atrophied at the affected spinal segment on the ipsilateral side (Hodges *et al.*, 2006). Cross-sectional area of the *multifidi* can be measured ultrasonographically. Individuals with back pain have significant asymmetry in left:right size of the *multifidi* compared to healthy asymptomatic subjects (Hides *et al.*, 2008) with muscular atrophy on the painful side of the back. Atrophy occurs within days, is selective for *multifidi* and does not involve other epaxial muscles (Danneels *et al.*, 2001). When the *multifidi* are inhibited they no longer stabilize the intervertebral joints in preparation for movement. The resulting instability may allow micromotion of the joints that predisposes to the development of further pathologies, such as osteoarthritis (Hides *et al.*, 1996). Even after the initial episode of back pain resolves, the *multifidi* remain dysfunctional and atrophied unless specific therapeutic exercises are performed (Hides *et al.*, 1996).

Horses with back pain seem to follow the same pattern as human patients. Severe osseous pathology has been associated with atrophy of ipsilateral *multifidi* at the same spinal level (Stubbs *et al.*, 2010). Thus ultrasonographic asymmetry of *multifidi* may be important as a diagnostic indicator that a horse currently has back pain or has had back pain in the past. It is reasonable to assume that the *multifidi* will not restore their size and function spontaneously, so special therapeutic exercises may be needed to activate and strengthen these muscles in order to restore their protective function in horses.

Therapeutic exercises that are effective for restoring function of the *multifidi* in people combine stability with mobility. It has been suggested that exercises that incorporate a static holding component between the concentric and eccentric phases of muscle contraction are most effective in restoring size of *multifidi* (Danneels *et al.*, 2001). The benefits of performing therapeutic exercises include a significant reduction in the risk of recurrence of back pain within 12 months from >80% to 30% (Hides *et al.*, 2001). In horses dynamic mobilization exercises are believed to be effective for activating and strengthening the muscles that move and stabilize the spine (Stubbs and Clayton, 2008). In a group of riding school horses that performed dynamic mobilization exercises regularly for 3 months, cross-sectional area of the *multifidi* increased on both the left and right sides at all six spinal levels that were evaluated (T10, T12, T14, T16, T18, L5). Furthermore, left:right symmetry of *multifidi* also improved at all 6 spinal levels (Stubbs *et al.*, 2011).

Core training for horses

One of the best ways to both prevent and to treat back pain in horses is through the regular use of core training exercises (Stubbs and Clayton, 2008). Dynamic mobilization exercises are a subset of the core training exercises that are used specifically to activate and strengthen the horse's core musculature. The term dynamic indicates that the horse is actively using his muscles to move his body. The term mobilization implies that the exercises require stretching and therefore have a suppling effect. However, we believe the main benefit of these exercises lies in their ability to stimulate the muscles that flex, bend and stabilize the spine.

In these exercises, the horse is taught to follow a controlled movement pattern using a bait (usually a carrot) or a target through a specific movement pattern that involves rounding and/or bending the neck and back. Rounding exercises move the chin to the horse's chest, between the knees, or between the fetlocks, a neck extension exercise stretches the neck forward, and bending exercises take the chin around to the side toward the girth, the flank, the hip, or the hock (Figure 2). In order to achieve and maintain these positions, the horse must move his neck to the required position while, at the same time, stabilizing his back and limbs to keep his balance. A large number of muscles are recruited. If you watch closely as a horse does the dynamic mobilization exercises, you can see contractions in the abdominal and back muscles, as well as the pelvic, hamstring and chest muscles.

Core strengthening exercises are a progression from the dynamic mobilization exercises. In these exercises pressure is applied to a specific anatomical area and the horse responds by rounding and/ or bending the spine. For example, pressure on the sternal midline

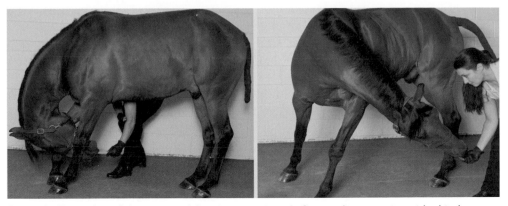

Figure 2. Examples of dynamic mobilization exercises. Left: rounding exercise with chin between carpi; right: lateral bending exercise with chin to tarsus. Note activation of abdominal, pelvic and hamstring muscles in the figure on the right.

results in rounding through the base of the neck, the withers and the saddle region. Pressure on the caudal vertebral spinous processes results in rounding of the caudal thoracic, lumbar and lumbosacral joints. Unilateral pressure to one side of the sacrocaudal region results in rounding and lateral bending. These exercises are described in detail in Stubbs and Clayton (2008).

Core training exercises should be used in young horses to activate the core musculature in preparation for ridden exercise. By strengthening these muscles prior to starting work under saddle, the horse is better able to cope with the effects of the rider's weight. It will also be easier for the rider to teach the horse to move with the back rounded during ridden exercise.

Core training exercises should be continued throughout the horse's career to maintain strength in the core muscles. When horses must be rested due to illness or injury, the exercises can usually be continued so that core strength is maintained and the core musculature will be strong when the horse returns to ridden exercise.

References

Danneels LA, Vanderstraeten GG, Cambier DC, Witvrouw EE, Bourgois J, Dankaerts W, De Cuyper HJ (2001) Effects of three different training modalities on the cross sectional area of the lumbar multifidus muscle in patients with chronic low back pain. Br J Sports Med 35:186-191.

Denoix JM (1998) Diagnosis of the cause of back pain in horses. Conf Eq Sports Med Sci. Pp 97-110.

Haussler KK (1999) Chiropractic Evaluation and Management. Vet Clin North Amer Eq Pract 15:195–208.

Haussler KK, Stover SM, Willits NH (1999) Pathologic changes in the lumbosacral vertebrae and pelvis in Thoroughbred racehorses. Am J Vet Res 60:143-153.

Hides J, Gilmore C, Stanton W, Bohlscheid E (2008) Multifidus size and symmetry among chronic LBP and healthy asymptomatic subjects. Manual Ther 13:43–49.

Hides JA, Jull GA, Richardson CA (2001) Long-term effects of specific stabilizing exercises for first-episode low back pain. Spine 26:E243-248.

Hides JA, Richardson CA, Jull GA (1996) Multifidus muscle recovery is not automatic after resolution of acute, first episode low back pain. Spine 21:2763-2769.

Hodges P, Holm AK, Hansson T, Holm S (2006) Rapid atrophy of the lumbar multifidus follows experimental disc or nerve root injury. Spine 31:2926-2933.

Stubbs NC, Clayton HM (2008) Activate your horse's core. Sport Horse Publications, Mason, MI.

Stubbs NC, Kaiser LJ, Hauptman J, Clayton HM (2011) Dynamic mobilization exercises increase cross sectional area of musculus multifidus. Eq Vet J. DOI: 10.1111/j.2042-3306.2010.00322.x

Stubbs NC, Riggs CM, Clayton HM, Hodges PW, Jeffcott LB, McGowan CM (2010) Spinal pathology and epaxial muscle ultrasonography in Thoroughbred racehorses. Eq Vet J 42 Suppl 38:654-661.

Equine nutrition – clinical cases where nutrition is involved

Manfred Coenen
Institut für Tierernährung, Ernährungsschäden und Diätetik, Veterinärmedizinische Fakultät, Universität Leipzig, Gustav-Kühn-Str. 8, 04159 Leipzig, Germany; coenen@vetmed.uni-leipzig.de

Feed and feeding are leading environmental factors that create direct or indirect impact on equine health. Horse owners/riders, trainers and veterinarians rank nutrition on the top regarding the role for health and performance. This general view on equine nutrition is contrasted in many cases by the daily care for feed quality and safe feeding management as well as by the effort to elaborate precise information on nutrition in case of low performance or disease in an individual horse or a group of horses. It should be noticed that animals do not respond to a mismatch in nutritional demands by visible changes in certain indicators. Even high performance horses can compensate defects in feed quality and nutrient supply without loosing their actual condition. Therefore, the absence of disease and/or of lack of performance is no proof for a safe nutrition and is no reason to not change the diet based on state of the art knowledge.

Demands for safe nutrition

A simple list characterizes basic needs for a diet:
1. covering requirements;
2. ingestible in terms of volume and palatability;
3. adequate regarding the specific conditions of digestion and metabolism;
4. good hygienic quality;
5. compatible with the individual;
6. safe regarding the quality of products (meat, milk);
7. minimizing impact on the environment.

Manfred Coenen

Covering requirements

The available scientific information about the energy and nutrient requirements ensures that there is no reason for health problems due to deficiencies or excesses. The bottleneck is the application of available data on requirements.

Feral horses or extensively ranged horses may have a suboptimal nutrient intake due to the available forage; this holds specifically for the protein, copper (Cu), zinc (Zn), selenium (Se) intake. However, the majority of equines are held under close human supervision or are even urbanized. These horses are faced by human driven decisions on nutrition which can override proven facts on requirements.

Examples of clinical relevance:
- mismatch of mineral provision to lactating mares on pasture;
- undesirable trace element and vitamin supply to performance horses;
- urolithiasis;
- trace element toxicosis;
- obesity.

Ingestible in terms of volume and palatability

A valuable estimate for the maximum rate of feed intake is 0.63 g DM min^{-1} kg BW$^{0.71}$ (DM = dry matter; BW = body weight); this figure is taken from an interspecies study including horses fed with fresh alfalfa (Shipley *et al.*, 1994). That means that the estimated rate of intake for a 500 kg horse is 52 g min^{-1}. Having access to poor pasture grass with 8 MJ digestible energy (DE) kg^{-1} DM a horse would need to ingest the feed at the max. rate of intake in ~2.6 h. In fact the horse will spend >12 h on feed intake. Consequently there is a huge difference between the minimum of time required for the intake and the normal behaviour related to feed ingestion. If feed is freely available the amount of ingested feed DM varies between ~55 (foals) and 150 (lactating mares) g DM kg BW$^{0.75}$ d^{-1}; 130-140 g DM kg BW$^{0.75}$ d^{-1} can be set for exercising horses. In conclusion, horses will consume feed DM >20 g kg^{-1} BW d^{-1}. Although the proportion of time spend for feed intake compared to the time available for feed exploration and selection has not been sufficiently well investigated it seems to be of minor relevance. The estimated DM intake of a 500 kg exercising horse is $\sim$14.3 kg d^{-1}. If the time for intake is restricted to 10 h d^{-1} the horse needs to ingest $\sim$ 1.4 kg DM h^{-1} = 24 g DM min^{-1}. This is far below the maximal rate of intake.

These data allow to conclude that:
- feed intake is not a limiting factor for high performance horses (in contrast to dairy cows) as long as feed is provided;
- loosing BW indicates:
  — a health problem;
  — or shortage in feed supply;
  — or straw as the only roughage.

Examples for clinical relevance: see next section.

Adequate regarding the specific conditions of digestion and metabolism

It needed surprisingly long time to become accepted that the gastro-intestinal tract (GIT) requires a specific architecture of the diet and communicates with the endocrine and central nervous system while processing the diet. The following facts make clear what is helpful to define the required dietary architecture:
- Saliva determines the intragastric environment.
- Saliva volume depends on chewing and chewing is simply the result of time for ingestion × chews/unit of time. The latter is remarkably constant ($\sim$1.5-1.8 Hz); the type of feed therefore determines saliva volume by the time for intake (e.g. 45 min kg^{-1} roughage vs. $\sim$10 min kg^{-1} grain).
- Cell wall constitution is dependent on:
  — speed of intake as well as the balance between gastric uptake and emptying;
  — passage rate in small intestine;
  — microbial activity in the entire GIT;
  — microbial digestion in the hindgut;
  — provision of products from microbial digestion:
    › water soluble vitamins;
    › volatile fatty acids;
  — nitrogen trapping in microbial protein;
  — intraintestinal water and electrolyte turnover.
- Mono-, disaccharides and starches depend on:

- the provision of monosaccharides (mainly glucose) to intermediary metabolism;
    - gut hormone responses;
    - insulin secretion.
- Hydrolysable carbohydrates (oligosaccharides, starches) can escape small intestinal decomposition and absorption:
    - due to their:
        › origin (ileo-caecal flow of starch [ICFS]: Corn > barley > oats);
        › processing (ICFS: native starch > mechanical > thermal starch processing);
        › quantity;
    - and result in:
        › lactic acid producing bacteria promotion;
        › depression of lactic acid consumers and cellulolytic acting bacteria;
        › loss of protozoa.

Fibrous feeds serve complex mechanisms of the GIT and are strictly linked to behaviour. Feeds high in non structural carbohydrates can counteract effects of fibre related carbohydrates and – in addition – induce endocrine responses that take immediate influence on target tissues like liver, muscle and adipose tissue. A minimum of structural carbohydrates and a maximum of non-structural carbohydrates have to be considered. Although several aspects have not been sufficiently well examined yet, a minimum of roughage has to be provided daily (balancing 100% of maintenance requirement in energy or minimum 20 g kg^{-1} BW d^{-1} [referring to 84-90% DM; equivalents for grass or ensiled products can be calculated in dependence on DM]) and a maximum of starch per meal (max. 1 g kg^{-1} BW meal^{-1}). These data can be used as guideline to prevent problems from the GIT, the behaviour of the horse and endocrine responses.

Examples of clinical relevance:
- abnormal behaviour (e.g. crip biting);
- damage of the gastric mucosa (EGUS);
- caecal dysfermentation;
- laminitis;
- low performance.

Good hygienic quality

Feed can not be and should not be a sterile substrate. A certain microbiota attached to the feed belongs to the normal quality. Organisms evaluated as specific pathogenic microbes are absent or negligible in the microbial community mentioned above. However, an elevated count of bacteria, moulds and yeasts indicates:
- risk for the feed:
  — spoilage – to be expected or existing already;
- risk for the animal:
  — by respirable particles;
  — ingestion of feed related microbes and their competition with the autochtone microbiota;
  — uptake of toxins of microbial origin:
    › bacterial toxins (e.g. toxins from *Clostridia* sp.);
    › mycotoxins (e.g. aflatoxin).

Toxicological events are impressive and characterized for the most important toxins but the mechanisms of damage in the GIT simply by elevated numbers of bacteria, moulds and yeasts are still not well understood. The definition of safe hygiene standards for feeds therefore is not based on experimental data like the upper safe level for Se but on data about the average quantity and quality of microbes on feed which are not incriminated to produce a health risk. Those data are available for most equine feeds and are an extremely helpful tool to perform risk assessment of a feeding condition.

Examples of clinical relevance:
- gastric tympany;
- spastic colic;
- hindgut tympany and/or displacement;
- toxicosis (mycotoxins, bacterial toxins).

Compatible with the individual

Individual horses may have individual set points to respond on a diet. The 'easy keeper' is a simple example. The genetic background, age history in nutrition and history of disease are major factors for a natural variation that requires adjusting a ration that is properly designed but not completely covering the needs of an individual horse. An undesirable feeding condition evaluated by body condition scoring and loss of performance are non-specific outcomes. A refusal of hay is a quite common event in some horses; up to now there is no satisfying explanation for this e.g. based on botanical composition.

The age-effect is mostly created by erosions of teeth or bad shape of teeth. The incomplete feed processing during intake results in a risk for GIT function and loss in feeding value. This can be associated with an age dependent loss on the availability of digestive enzymes and in gut motility.

In the case of a disease there can be an extra need for a nutrient. Most diseases related to infections are linked to elevated energy and protein metabolism and turnover respectively. There is no model to create factors for corrections of diets to consider the side effects of disease. A loss of fluids from a wound can result in high protein loss and a drop in plasma protein fractions.

The stress of disease includes a challenge for antioxidative capabilities of the organism; little is known about the effects e.g. chronic pulmonary dysfunction on antioxidative systems. However it has been shown in ruminants that antioxidative support after treating a displaced abomasum enhances postsurgical recovery. Case orientated feed selection, feed processing and dosing as well as selected nutrients for enforced supply are sufficient countermeasures.

The principles for the adaptation of a diet for an individual horse can be summarized as follows:
- in the case of feed refusal:
  — change feed;
  — moisten feed;
  — add some oil;
  — pelleted feed;
- consider age:
  — roughage processing (cubes);
  — thermal grain processing;
  — selection of carrots or sugar beet pulp;
  — addition of oil (max 1 ml kg^{-1} BW d^{-1});
  — 25% of protein requirement in addition to proteins of high quality;

- side effects of disease:
  - balance specific needs for disabled organs (e.g. renal insufficiency);
  - avoid off feed periods;
  - adjust energy and protein supply:
    - › preference of thermally processed grain;
    - › add protein of high quality;
  - ensure intake of carotine, vitamin E, copper, zinc, selenium at the recommended level for high performance horses;
  - feed the microbiota of the GIT (carrots, sugar beet pulp, brewers yeast).

Examples of clinical relevance:
- wound infection;
- chronic inflammation;
- repeated episodes of colic;
- specific dysfunctions of certain tissues/organs (e.g. kidney, liver, skin, muscle, bone);
- weight loss;
- loose faeces;
- insufficient chewing in aged horses.

Safe regarding the quality of products (meat, milk)

The use of horse meat for human consumption requires the consideration of the same security measures as for other food producing animals (e.g. utilisation of drugs). The protein of meat cannot be influenced by nutrition as far as in general there is no deficit of amino acids. However, the fat:protein ratio can be influenced by diets high in energy but limited in protein.

More important is the impact of nutrition on milk composition regarding the primary use for the foal or the secondary utilisation by humans as specific dietary ingredient or for other purposes. The trace element and vitamin intake of the mare is partially reflected by milk.

It should be noted that covering the requirements of the lactating mare ensures proper milk composition and enforced nutrients in the diet of mares does not provide benefits.

Examples for clinical relevance: rare

Minimizing impact on the environment

The negative impact of horse feeding practice on the environment has become a matter of concern. Oversupply of protein and minerals results in elevated faecal or renal excretion and transfer of nitrogen, macro and trace elements to the soil. In addition, volatile compounds may be liberated; ammonia is the most relevant. Provision of nutrients adjusted to the requirements ensures keeping the emissions from horse husbandry within an acceptable range.

Reasons for a non-safe diet & feeding routine

The major reasons are due to:
1. wrong feed selection and dosing;
2. disadvantageous feed processing;
3. risks created by feeding technique;
4. contamination of feeds:
   — biotic;
   — non-biotic contamination.

Most nutrition related health problems are related to one or more of the following causes:

■ Hay with 35% crude fibre in dry matter is suitable for horses at maintenance level but not for performance horses. The critical point in practice is simply the lack of objective information on feed composition. Roughage should represent a minimum of 60% of dietary dry matter, in most cases ~80%. It is evident that information about this part of the ration is a leading factor. If missed, concentrate selection in particular for high performance horses remains imprecise or even risky.

■ The quantity of roughage is a problem of first order in feeding practice (see points 1-3 above). Diets low in hay reduce the effect of unknown chemical composition of the entire diet because concentrate (e.g. grain) is more uniform or has been even analyzed. This 'bad feed' dosing impacts the behaviour of horses and induces alternative strategies for the horse to be more entertained e.g. by increasing straw consumption.

■ The use of supplements needs to be the result of a ration calculation. Many mineral feeds are used without precise rationing. The result is an unbalanced macro element supply (e.g. Ca-intake at 3fold of requirement) but still marginal Zn-intake.

■ The use of supplements often negates scientific data on requirements and efficiency (e.g. enforced Fe-supplementation which is at least useless).

The aims of processing feed are to:

■ improve digestibility (e.g. starch digestibility by thermal processing);

■ ensure intake;

■ inhibit separation of ingredients;

■ improve stability (e.g. small surface of pelleted feed vs. coarse feed);

■ compensate specific behaviour of feed architecture during intake (e.g. volume expansion of pelleted sugar beet pulp).

The feeding technique is directed to ensure intake (e.g. in a herd), to limit the rate of intake and to maintain safe gastric function. No roughage at night will speed up concentrate ingestion at the following morning. This is associated with low saliva production and challenges gastric function. The load of the stomach by feed is of special interest in case of discontinuous pasturing. A starchy meal before turnout of the horses on pasture predisposes the animal to become affected by dysfermentation and uncontrolled gas production in the stomach.

An often neglected aspect in feeding technique is the stimulation of compensatory straw intake if hay is low in quantity or badly distributed over meals with long intermeal periods. This can increase the risk for colic by impaction.

The contamination of feeds fits with point 4 in the first section. The strong link between dust levels in stables and feed quality explains the need for feed evaluation regarding the hygiene standard. This aspect of feed quality is an issue for GIT function. It is of great interest that after challenging exercise the defence capabilities of the respiratory tract are severely depressed and the small intestine may show a reduced integrity. The mechanisms on how the intestinal tract is affected by bacteria and moulds is not clear (s. first section); the phagocytosis in the respiratory tract obviously is becoming overridden while in the gut the interaction with the physiological microbiota and the communication with the gut wall and associated compounds like serotonin is still a matter to be scrutinized.

As mentioned above, microbial toxins can induce intestinal and extra intestinal damages. Toxins from *Clostridia* and some moulds are of practical relevance. As mycotoxins are naturally ubiquitous occurring substances, they are detectable in many cases. It needs a specific evaluation of the detected toxin regarding type and concentration in order to define the risk level.

Conclusion

Basic guidelines that define safe nutrition are needed to check the equine diet to reduce or even avoid feed or feeding related health and behavioural risks. In many cases nutrition is not the only driving force for a disease but risk assessment and avoidance requires the management of nutritional factors.

References

Shipley LA, Gross JE, Spalinger DE, Hobbs NT, Wunder BA (1994) The scaling of intake rate in mammalian herbivores. Am Nat 143:1055-1082.

Feeding and training the endurance horse: how science can serve the practitioners

Anne-Gaëlle Goachet and Véronique Julliand
URANIE-USC 'Nutrition of the Athletic Horse', AgroSup Dijon, 26 bvd Dr.
Petitjean, BP 87999, 21079 Dijon cedex, France; ag.goachet@agrosupdijon.fr

How researchers in equine nutrition came to train endurance horses

Our AgroSup Dijon research team aims at improving the feeding energy system for exercised horses. That means defining more precisely feeding recommendations in terms of energetic nutrition for those horses that are in the real world of training and competition. To reach that goal, the need for other equine models than horses at maintenance soon arose and we created an experimental endurance equestrian team. This is how doing research led us to manage endurance equine athletes.

This story started ten years ago when Anne-Gaëlle Goachet joined our research group as a young student in agricultural engineering. At that time, we were conducting experimental trials to better understand the impact of feeding practices on the digestibility of dietary energetic constituents and on the microbial balance of the hindgut ecosystem. However, because our horses were at maintenance, we could not feed them athletic horses' diets. For instance, our sedentary horses' intakes were lower than those of trained horses, bringing non-comparable data in terms of digestion. This limited the application of our nutritional observations towards the exercised horse. Anne-Gaëlle Goachet, as an endurance rider keen on completing a PhD on equine nutrition, saw here a unique opportunity to combine both her passion and her work and offered to start an experimental endurance horses team. This project looked feasible as it did not require specific animal facilities, but 'only' good horses, good riders and good training tracks and grounds. As head of the research team, Véronique Julliand, subscribed to that challenge and shared with Anne-Gaëlle Goachet the set-up of a new research project about the impact of endurance conditioning on the digestion. Luckily we obtained the major support of Marcel Mézy, a French breeder of Arabian horses, who accepted to leave six of his horses to us in our animal facilities. Also, we had both a pool of good riders among the Agrosup students, and the support of our general director. In September 2002, the AgroSup endurance team was born.

From there, our experimental endurance team served as a support for many research projects: one PhD, three Master research projects and a one-year collaborative project with French and Belgium colleagues. We generated many data regarding the nutrition of the endurance horse which was our scientific objective. Because our horses were kept under experimental conditions, we recorded lots of observations. This allowed us to generate also many 'by-products' regarding the management of endurance horses during training and also during competition, such as for instance feeding, training program, shoeing of the horses. The present paper aims at sharing what science brought to us and could be of interest for people involved in equestrian endurance.

The AgroSup endurance team: horses and performance

From 2002 to 2010, 23 horses were accommodated and trained in our animal facilities: 8 mares and 15 geldings (Table 1). Most of them were pure-bred Arabians, only one being cross-bred Arabian. Their height ranged from 149 to 160 cm, and was 153 ± 3 cm in average. Their average body weight (BW) was 434 ± 25 kg, with the lightest and heaviest horses weighing 361 ± 5 kg and 512 ± 15 kg respectively (Table 1). Height and BW ranged within typical values observed in Arabian horses (Pietrzak and Strzelec, 2002; Métayer *et al.*, 2003; Barnes *et al.*, 2010). At arrival, horses were adult, but relatively young: 16 were less than seven years old (Table 1). Only half of the horses had experienced endurance training prior to their arrival. Three mares, Naya, Samira and Bemira, were not broken, being broodmares for several years before entering our team.

Horses were selected according to three main criteria: breed, physical characteristics, and, if any, anterior performances in

Table I. Agro Sup Dijon endurance horses.

Name	Breed	Parents (stallion*mare)	Sex[1]	Height cm	Weight kg	Age (years)		Endurance level	
						At arrival	At departure	At arrival	At departure
Jeffka de Champolot	Arabian	Nisscusko*Banika	G	154	425±6	5	6	60 km	60 km
Dar Es Salam	Arabian	Menfouk*Karina II	G	154	361±5	10	11	90 km	90 km
Djid de Bozouls	Arabian	Prim de Syrah*Djella de Bozouls	G	155	428±11	5	9	(Leisure)	160 km
Djel de Bozouls	Arabian	Rim*Idjella	G	152	439±14	6	10	(Leisure)	90 km
Rim	Arabian	Diaf*Aiffa Lotoise	G	152	434±14	10	14	60 km	90 km
Shalikhan	Arabian	Agan Khan*Shalimar Bintpandi	G	157	435±10	6	7	(Jumping)	60 km
Samira de Bozouls	Arabian	Rim*Shaa	F	153	415±20	6	7	(Breeding)	20 km
Djerifa de Bozouls	Arabian	Prim de Syrah*Djerba de Bozouls	F	154	432±9	4	7	(Flat racing)	90 km
Bemira de Bozouls	Arabian	Diaf*Benamira	F	154	421±14	5	8	(Breeding)	130 km
Naya de Bozouls	Arabian	Rim*Nadia Al S gour	F	149	443±14	6	13	(Breeding)	160 km
Djourba de Bozouls	Arabian	Prim de Syrah*Djerba de Bozouls	F	156	446±10	7	8	(Flat racing)	60 km
Ziza de Bozouls	Arabian	Prim de Syrah*Zaara de Bozouls	F	149	425±12	10	11	130 km	130 km
Djour de Bozouls	Arabian	Prim de Syrah*Djerba de Bozouls	G	153	429±12	5	8	40 km	90 km
Zaaf de Bozouls	Arabian	Prim de Syrah*Zaara de Bozouls	G	152	444±14	4	11	(Flat racing)	160 km
Naid de Bozouls	Arabian	Prim de Syrah*Nadia Al Sigour	G	155	463±14	7	9	90 km	130 km

Table I. Continued.

Name	Breed	Parents (stallion*mare)	Sex[1]	Height cm	Weight kg	Age (years)		Endurance level	
						At arrival	At departure	At arrival	At departure
Nazia de Niellans	Arabian	Mabrouck HN*Fara Bint Naalia	F	155	438±9	7	8	90 km	160 km
Kebar de Jalima	Arabian	Nichem*Azzra	G	153	384±14	11	14	130 km	130 km
Belik de Jalima	Arabian	Piruet*Laiocha	G	153	418±11	10	13	130 km	130 km
Halan Le Texan	Cross-Bred Arabian	Bajou*Texane	G	160	512±15	13	14	130 km	130 km
Siglavy Bagdady Bibor	Shagya Arabian	Lajosmizse Siglavy Bagdad *Shagya Boldogsog 1462	F	148	388±7	13	14	90 km	130 km
Nafar des Agachiols	Arabian	Farid del Saul*Naya de Bozouls	G	150	458±14	7	9	(Pasture)	130 km
Riminita de Bozouls	Arabian	Rim*Nadia Al Sigour	F	150	423±11	13	14	160 km	130 km
Assidaroi de Bozouls	Arabian	Farid del Saul*Assida de Bozouls	G	151	453±9	6	7	(Pasture)	40 km

[1] F: female; G: geldings.

endurance. Arabians or Arabian crosses were chosen as they are the most competitive horses in endurance events (Crandell, 2005; Cerchiaro *et al.*, 2004; Liesens, 2009). Due to muscular, metabolic and morphological predispositions, Arabians are better adapted to endurance work compared to other breeds. Their specific muscle fibre composition (Lopez-Rivero *et al.*, 1991) allows them superior oxidative capacity. Their energetic metabolism is particularly adapted to endurance exercise (Prince *et al.*, 2002). And also their conformational and locomotor profile increases their endurance ability: they are small and thin, with a short back, an inclined pelvis, open haunch and closed hock (Métayer *et al.*, 2003) which allows an efficient running economy (Cottin *et al.*, 2010). As lameness is the first cause of elimination in endurance events (69% of all eliminations in FEI elite endurance rides; Burger and Dollinger, 1998; Nagy *et al.*, 2010), our second criteria was the soundness and straightness of legs and feet. When horses had already experienced endurance rides, we did not select them if they had been eliminated for lameness. Contrary to common practice, we did not take into account the cardiac recovery power in our selection criteria.

By definition, 'endurance riding is a competition to test the competitor's ability to safely manage the stamina and fitness of the horse over an endurance course in a competition over the track, the distance, the climate, the terrain and the clock. The competition consists of a number of phases. No phase may exceed 40 km and should, in principle, be not less than 20 km in length. At the end of each phase, there will be a compulsory halt for veterinary inspection. The combination that finishes the course in the shortest time will be classified as the winner of the competition after successfully completing all final Veterinary Inspections and medication control as well as other protocols in place for the safety of the horse and rider' (www.fei.org). In total, our horses competed in 108 rides, from 20 to 160 km, registered in FFE (Fédération Française d'Equitation) and FEI (Fédération Equestre Internationale) endurance events. According to the qualification procedure required by the FFE and the FEI rules, they had to successfully complete one ride of 20 km, one ride of 40 km, one ride of 60 km and two rides of 90 km to be eligible to participate to elite level rides (130 and 160 km in one day). Over the 108 rides, 40 rides were from 20 to 60 km, 29 rides of 90 km; 34 were 2 stars CEI, and 5 were 3 stars CEI. That represented something like

9,500 km! To complete a ride, one horse has to pass all the veterinary inspections and examinations, before, during (vet-gates) and at the end of the ride, and to demonstrate its fitness to continue. Fitness is evaluated by pulse recovery, metabolic stability and gait (www.fei.org; www.ffe.com). We got a global completion rate of 80%, which is in accordance with results observed in French endurance rides (Burger and Dollinger, 1998). This completion rate differed according to the competition level: for 20, 40 and 60 km rides, it was 100%, which is very close to the results from the last four years of FFE endurance events data (superior to 90%); it was 79%, 65 and 60% for 90 km 130 km events and 160 km events respectively, which was close to those obtained from European and international surveys and data analysis (Burger and Dollinger, 1998; Robert *et al.*, 2002; Meyrier, 2003; Munoz *et al.*, 2006; Nagy *et al.*, 2010), where it ranged from 40 to 67%. Under field conditions, many horses are able to compete 20, 40 and 60-km endurance events, without a specific individual capacity, training or feeding programme, while performing in 90-km level races and above is more selective. These data suggest that the endurance effort really begins from 90 km rides on.

When our horses did not complete the race, it was mostly due to elimination for lameness (55%) and retirement by the rider (36%) (Table 2). Lameness concerned the forelegs (8 of 12 cases) mainly and hind legs in a lesser extent, as observed by Meyrier (2003). Elimination for metabolic reasons concerned only one horse (9%), which was eliminated because he did not recover pulse within the time, the first time at the final inspection of a 90 km ride, and the second time at the recovery check of the third loop of a 130 km ride. This horse did not require medical treatment to recover. These results are representative for elimination causes in endurance rides (Robert *et al.*, 2002; Meyrier, 2003; Nagy *et al.*, 2010) and confirm that locomotion is the major limiting factor in endurance.

Depending on the duration of our experiments, and also according to their performances (too low or on the contrary, too high), horses stayed from one to seven years at AgroSup, on average two years and a half. Four horses, Dar Es Salam, Djerifa de Bozouls, Bemira de Bozouls and Djid de Bozouls, were bought and joined elite endurance stables in UAE and Bahrein. After having being trained at AgroSup from 2004 to 2006,

Table 2. Agro Sup Dijon horses' results in 130 and 160 km endurance events.

Year	Location	Distance	Entered	Qualified	Completion rate (%)	Winner speed (km/h)	Horse	Result	Speed (km/h)
2005	Neris Les Bains	130	81	45	56	16.9	Naya de Bozouls	Lameness VG 4	-
	Le Pertre	130	99	53	54	19.3	Bemira de Bozouls	31	15.3
2006	Ribiers	130	122	70	57	18.6	Naya de Bozouls	64	13.4
	St Galmier	160	81	31	38	18.62	Naya de Bozouls	21	14.1
	Oletta	2*60	93	50	54	17.4	Zaaf de Bozouls	Lameness VG2	-
	Nancy	130	74	34	46	15.7	Djid de Bozouls	29	13.1
							Djel de Bozouls	Metabolic VG3	-
							Rim	Retired by the rider VG2	-
2007	Néris Les Bains	130	85	55	65	17.3	Djel de Bozouls	Lameness VG1	-
	Compiègne	130	108	55	52	18.3	Zzaf de Bozouls	36	16.1
	St Galmier	130	80	55	70	20	Naya de Bozouls	23	18.9
2008	Monpazier	130	105	61	58	16.5	Naya de Bozouls	Lameness VG3	-
							Naid de Bozouls	Lameness VG2	-
							Kebar de Jalima	32	14.6
							Bibor	Lameness VG3	-
	Mons	130	42	25	60	18.7	Zaaf de Bozouls	16	15.1
							Nazia de Niellans	15	15.1
							Belik de Jalima	14	15.1
	St Galmier	130	81	56	69	21.0	Zaaf de Bozouls	32	16.9
							Nazia de Niellans	Lameness VG3	16.9
							Halan Le Texan	30	16.9
	Vittel	130	63	37	59	17.9	Naya de Bozouls	10	15.7
							Naid de Bozouls	23	14.7
							Kebar de Jalima	24	14.7

Table 2. Continued.

Year	Location	Distance	Entered	Qualified	Completion rate (%)	Winner speed (km/h)	Horse	Result	Speed (km/h)
2009	Argentan	130	27	22	81	18.3	Belik de Jalima	11	16.5
							Riminita de Bozouls	12	16.5
	Chavanay	130	44	15	34	17.3	Zaaf de Bozouls	4	15.6
							Kebar de Jalima	Lameness VG3	-
	Compiègne	130	90	46	51	21.0	Kebar de Jalima	30	17.8
							Nafar de Agachiols	43	15.6
	Le Pertre	130	46	26	57	18.5	Belik de Jalima	8	16.8
							Riminita de Bozouls	12	16.6
	Monpazier	130	96	40	42	18.3	Naya de Bozouls	3	17.3
							Zaaf de Bozouls	Lameness VG3	-
	Vittel	130	37	23	62	16.3	Naya de Bozouls	2	16.2
2010	Florac	160	155	64	41	17.6	Zaaf de Bozouls	42	14.4
	Monpazier	160	21	13	62	18.3	Naya de Bozouls	5	17.1
	Rambouillet	160	52	28	54	17.3	Belik de Jalima	Lameness VG1	-
							Nafar des Agachiols	Retired by the rider VG3	-

Djour de Bozouls was enrolled in the French national endurance team and participated at the 2009 European Championship (Assisi, Italy).

The management of our endurance horses in training

When our AgroSup endurance team started on September 2002, six Arabian horses joined our animal facilities. At that time, we had no specific equipment for sport horses but we gradually purchased the basics for riding. Two years later, our research team moved into more convenient facilities. On October 2006, we moved again and became established in brand new facilities which we had largely contributed to build in accordance with our specific needs. Today these facilities can accommodate up to twenty sport horses and have individual paddocks, and an automatic horse walker. In addition, these facilities are located in a very hilly countryside, which offers better training tracks compared to the plain ground we had before. Because we experienced all these different environments, we were able to make some comparisons.

Housing

In many countries, the majority of endurance horses are maintained in pasture or in a stall with access to pasture (Nieto *et al.*, 2004; Marguet, 2009). However, when our horses arrived at AgroSup in 2002, we only had a stable with individual free stalls, but no turn-out. Except when they were ridden, horses were maintained in stalls, and because of the confinement, they became nervous and very difficult to train in outdoor tracks, which was really insecure for riders and horses. When we moved to the next stable, we had the opportunity to build individual paddocks which allowed to turn-out horses all day long. Thus, they became calmer and worked a lot better. Managing horses in individual paddocks rather than in collective ones enabled to avoid injuries among horses that could compromise performances and to monitor water and feed intake individually.

Training

Few data are available regarding training strategies for endurance. The training programs we applied were established from our personal experience combined with the advices of endurance trainers: Julien Goachet, who spent several years in UAE endurance stables, and Jean-Louis Leclerc, who was the trainer and selector of the French endurance team from 2005 to 2010. From 2002 to 2010, the daily monitoring of exercise (date, rider, and duration of exercise...) allowed us to determine a posteriori the training programs we had applied to prepare the horses for 60, 90 and 130 km. The training season should theoretically match competitive season which takes place between March and October in France. In practice, our start was delayed due to the cold climate during winter in our region. As the outdoor tracks were frozen and slippery, our training program could not start before March-April. So our horses had a resting period from December to March-April, and began competition in June.

Three different kinds of exercises

Outdoor rides: contrary to other equestrian sports where horses are trained on racetracks or in arenas (Clayton, 1991; Authié, 2009), endurance training happens outdoor with rides in trails. In accordance with field practices in France (Leclerc, 2009; Liesens, 2009), we choose a duration of two hours on average for these outdoor rides. From 2002 to 2006, horses were trained in very flat areas and outdoor rides were mainly at trot at 14 km/h, and with approximately 20% walk at 6 km/h, and 10% gallop at 20 km/h. From 2006, the countryside was a lot hillier with very hard grounds. Then, the average training ride comprised a lot more walk (80%), and only 15% trot plus 5% gallop. Consequently, the average exercise speed decreased from 13 to 8 km/h. The distance of the rides was 12 km at least and 30 km at most (Figure 1). According to the stage of training, the hills were climbed at walk (at the beginning of the training season), or at trot, in order to increase exercise intensity. Horses always went down the hill walking in order to avoid tendon and joint injuries. During outdoor rides, horses spent 55% of the time working at heart rate (HR) between 80 and 110 bpm. Physiologically, these outdoor rides can be classified as long-lasting endurance exercises (Bergero *et al.*, 2005). The outdoor ride efforts were less intense than event efforts (performed mainly within 110 and 130 bpm; Figure 2), being so safer for the legs.

Canters on racetrack: these canter exercises aimed at working at higher speed and intensity than the outdoor rides. Two hours canters

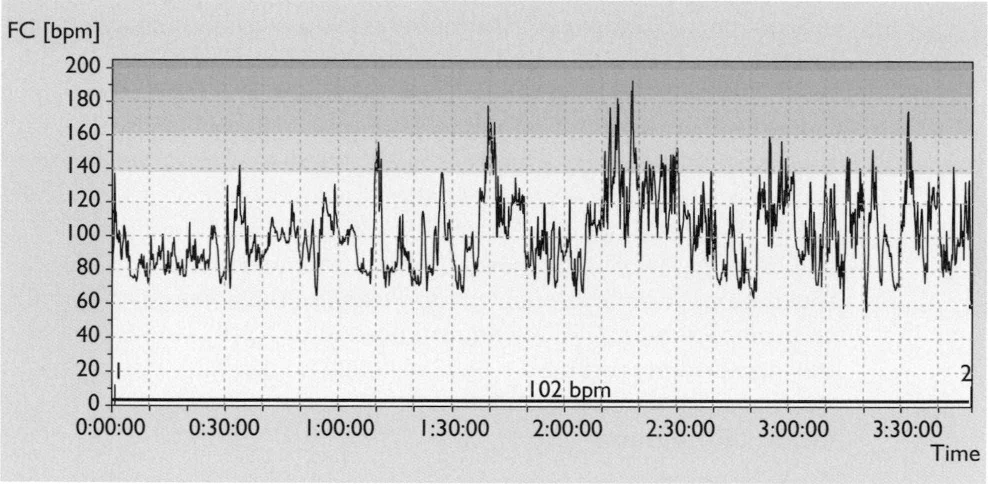

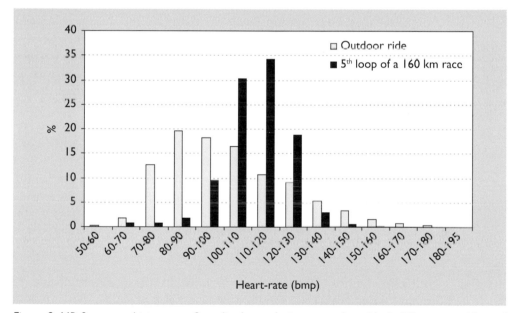

Figure 1. Recorded HR of an elite horse during a 30 km training session, in hilly countryside.

Figure 2. HR frequency histogram of an elite horse during an outdoor ride, in hilly countryside, and the 5th loop of a 160-km ride.

at 18-20 km/h were included in the training program, only for horses preparing 130 and 160 km events. These exercises were done within the last month and two weeks minimum before the competition. As recommended by Leclerc (2009), canters were done on racetracks, and not on hard surfaces, in order to limit concussions and avoid joint injuries.

Horse walker: as there is limited scientific data about the use and the potential benefits of horse walker (Parkins, 2009), we followed professional trainers' recommendations and field practices. Our horses were walked one hour at 7 km/h five days a week, 3 months prior to and all along the training period, in addition (and not substitution) of the basal training. This enabled us to exercise the horses earlier in the endurance season, (i.e. in January instead of April), and to increase the workload per week from 6h45 to 10h00 hours (Table 3).

Training programs

According to Clayton (1991), in the early years of conditioning, competitions are incorporated into the conditioning schedule when the horse reaches an appropriate level of fitness, and they are regarded as a part of the conditioning process rather than an end in themselves. On the other hand, an experienced endurance horse is prepared for specific races each year, and the annual conditioning program is planned so that the horse reaches peak fitness at these predetermined times.

Generally, our un-experienced horses competed in 20, 40 and 60 km rides in the first season of training, and in two 90-km races the second year of training. After two years of conditioning at minimum, our horses were able to compete in elite levels. At those levels, horses were prepared to compete in two races per year on average. The training programs were different depending on whether the horse was un-experienced or experienced.

Training for 20, 40 and 60 km rides: at these lower stages of competition, horses were ridden twice a week, during 1h30 and 2h30 hours, with a relatively low weekly workload (Table 3). Horses did not complete canters on racetracks and were not exercised in the walker. A posteriori, we counted 12 weeks of training on average to prepare horses to compete in 20, 40, 60 km endurance rides.

Training for 90 km rides: to prepare horses for 90 km rides, exercise type and frequency was similar to the training program for 20, 40 and

Table 3. Training programs applied to prepare horses for different levels of competition.

		Training program for 20, 40 and 60 km rides	Training program for 90 km rides	Training program for 130 and 160 km rides	
		2004-2005	2006-2007	2008	2009
Countryside		Flat	Flat	Hilly	Hilly
Outdoor rides	Frequency (per week)	2.0	2.0	3.0	2.3
	Duration (hours)	1h45	2h15	2h15	2h15
	Speed (km/h)	13	13	8	8
Walker	Frequency (per week)	-	-	-	5
	Duration (hours)	-	-	-	1h00
	Speed (km/h)	-	-	-	7
Canter	Frequency	-	-	3 weeks before a race	3 weeks before a race
	Duration (hours)	-	-	2h00	2h00
	Speed (km/h)	-	-	18-20	18-20
Total workload per week (hours)		3h30	4h30	6h45	10h00
Training period (weeks)		12	19	20	20

60 km rides, except that the duration of the rides increased to 2h15 on average. Consequently the weekly workload increased to 4h30 instead of 3h30 (Table 3). The training period was of 19 weeks.

Training for 130 and 160 km: for the highest levels of competitions, we used two different training programs with or without the walker. In both programs, canters were added before the events, and exercise frequency increased compared to the lower stages of training. This significantly impacted the total workload, which was 6h45 without walker and up to 10h00 with the walker (Table 3). With both programs, 20 weeks of training were necessary to prepare horses for 130 and 160 events.

Feeding

The feeding program of our endurance horses changed over the years and probably improved as we went along and accumulated experience. The first year, we set the ratio forage/concentrate at 60/40 on a dry matter (DM) basis. This was the ratio we used previously for our experimental horses. Because we wanted our horses to receive at least 8 kg hay per day, the quantity of pelleted feed was 5.5 kg per day and the total ingestion level reached 2.8% BW. Hay was given in two equal meals at 10:00 and 16:00 and pelleted feed in two equal meals at 08:00 and 17:30. Theoretically, this ration covered the nutritional needs recommended by INRA for horses providing a moderate exercise (INRA, 1984), as our horses were trained to compete in 90 km rides. However, our horses gained weight and body condition score. They looked nervous and one even developed muscular pathology resembling rhabdomyolysis, probably due to the high amount of concentrate they were fed. We thus decided to readjust our rations by increasing the ratio forage/concentrate, keeping a high dry matter intake, and to use BW and BCS as monitoring tools instead of INRA recommendations. On average, our horses received approximately 10 kg DM of hay daily, whatever the training level. The daily supply of concentrate increased progressively from 1 to 2.4 kg DM per horse and per day with training in order to maintain optimal BW and BCS. On average, the level of feed intake varied from 2.5 to 2.9% BW, and hay represented at least 80% of the total DM intake. This is in complete agreement with feeding practices commonly reported in the field (Ralston, 1988; Crandell, 2005, 2010), and represents probably the specificity of endurance horse feeding, in contrast to other equestrian disciplines, such as flat racing (Gallagher *et al.*, 1992), eventing (Burk and Williams, 2008), or jumping (Valle *et al.*, 2009). The hay we fed our horses was first-cut meadow hay, providing an average digestible energy of 2 Mcal/kg DM which corresponds to 0.5 UFC/kg DM (Table 4). We are aware that whatever the level of training, it is essential to provide large quantities of good quality forages to endurance horses. It ensures the behavioural integrity of the animal (Nicol, 2000; Goodwin *et al.*, 2001 cited by Geor, 2005) as well as the optimal health of its hindgut microbial ecosystem (Julliand and Ralston, 2006) which largely contributes to the energetic supply of the animal. Thanks to the fibrolytic communities inhabiting the hindgut, the horse can take advantage of the cell-wall polysaccharides that are broken down by enzymes excreted by the micro-organisms into sugars that are then hydrolyzed and lead to the formation of Volatile Fatty Acids (VFA). The VFA solely produced in the cecum have been reported to provide an average of 30% of the total energetic allowances in equine (Glinsky *et al.*, 1976). Moreover forages contribute to increase the water consumption and also the function as a fluid and electrolyte reservoir of the equine hindgut (Meyer *et al.*, 1987; Danielsen *et al.*, 1995; Warren *et al.*, 2001) which is very useful for endurance horses having high fluid losses during competition. Also, the physical presence of fiber in the digestive system will help maintain the blood flow to the gut tissue during exercise and could prevent colic (Duren, 1998). Our horses had free access to a salt block and did not receive any other supplement. They also had free access to water and drank in average 25 l per day.

The management of our endurance horses in competition

For the purpose of one experiment run by Stéphanie Zentz, a Master student in 2009, we monitored the BW, the BCS, the feed and water intake of six horses before, during and after the 130 km race which data will be partly reported here.

Housing

Whereas horses were transported to the event place the day of the race for the lower levels of competition (20, 40, and 60 km), they arrived

Table 4. Composition of hay and concentrate used at AgroSup Dijon.

	Hay							Concentrate		
	2004	2005	2006	2007	2008	2009	2010	2004-2007	2008	2009-2010
Producer								Royal Horse	SA Etienne	DP Nutrition
Commercial name								Horse Prim pellets	Olympic pellets	DP Puissance pellets
DM	87.9	87.7	86.8	87.5	88.8	90.4	92.5	89.9	89.8	88.0
CP	-	-	-	-	-	7.3	7.6	11.5	12.2	12.5
Starch	-	-	-	-	-	-	-	21.0	23.0	18.0
Ash	5.2	5.5	7.2	6.5	6.8	6.7	7.4	8.4	8.7	7.4
Fat	0.9	1.2	1.3	1.0	-	-	-	2.2	3.7	3.5
NDF	66.9	60.4	65.2	58.2	63.9	65.9	62.7	39.8	33.2	40.1
ADF	35.8	34.4	36.4	33.2	33.4	35.8	37.5	21.1	16.7	17.2
ADL	5.1	5.6	5.1	3.9	4.4	4.3	6.1	4.8	3.9	3.4
UFC/kg DM	0.51	0.55	0.49	0.55	0.51	0.50	0.50	0.85	0.90	0.90
Mcal DE/kg DM	2.06	2.22	2.02	2.23	2.08	2.02	2.05	2.91	3.15	3.22

DM: dry matter; CP: crude protein; NDF: neutral detergent fiber; ADF: acid detergent fiber; ADL: acid detergent lignin; UFC: Unité Fourragère Cheval; DE: Digestible Energy.

several days (3 days) before the race for higher levels of competition (90 km and more). Individual stalls with straw bedding were offered by the event organizer but we choose to keep our horses on artificial bedding as usual, in order to avoid excessive ingestion of straw. Also, we wanted them to have access to paddock and free exercise on the event place, in order to avoid muscular problems (exertional rhabdomyolysis) during the race. If there was no possibility to build paddocks, our horses were walked in hand or ridden at walk.

Shoeing

To our knowledge, there are no data reported on the type of shoes used for endurance horses. This is why we conformed to field practices in France. If regular steel shoes were used for training, a specific shoeing was necessary for competitions, especially for 90 or longer km events. In endurance, shoeing has to take into account the duration of exercise and the trails' characteristics. Except in Gulf countries, where rides are run faster, a 130 km ride last between 6 and 10 hours, and a 160 km ride between 8 and 13 hours in many countries (www.atrm.com). Also, characteristics of the ground can vary a lot, according to area and climate. Sometimes our horses had to run on very hard surfaces as asphalt, on stony tracks, or on slippery surfaces, as wet grass-covered tracks. That is why as recommended by Pelissier (2009), we chose shoeing being comfortable and light, absorbent, non-slip, protective, solid and durable, that should maintain the horse proprioception. Then, the running shoes we used for our horses had an important rolling on the external front border to ease the process of break over in front feet (Van Heel *et al.*, 2006) and wide coverage thanks to wide branches to protect the sole. Depending on the nature of the track, we selected shoes in steel or in aluminium. Aluminium was used for many events because it's lighter than steel, and reduces the fatigue (Benoît *et al.*, 1993). However, steel was chosen in some cases, especially for races on stony tracks (Florac for example), as it is more resistant than aluminium. Hoof pads were used to improve shock absorption and avoid concussion (Benoit *et al.*, 1993). Contrary to the leather pads used in many other equestrian disciplines (O'Grady, 2008), the pads used in endurance are of polyurethane (Pelissier, 2009). The technical properties of these pads depend on their thickness, weight, and density (simple or bi-density pad). We had the opportunity to use different pads, as the regular Shock Tamer pads (full flat pad covering the entire sole, 4,5 mm, dual density), the MV2 dynamic enduro (80 g, 3 mm, dual density), and the blue plastic pads (115 g, 3 mm, simple density). Packing materials (ultra-soft silicone) were also used to fill the hollow between the sole and the pad to avoid sand, earth or stone intrusion. As recommended by Pelissier (2009), packing materials have to be as soft as possible (10 shore D) to avoid any pressure on the sole. However, we had some horses having highly sensitive sole, flat hoofs or being long-pasterned that did not support any pressure on the sole, getting lame after being shoed with pads and silicone. For those horses, the farrier cut the pads in V-notched to keep the frog exposed, or opened the pad on the toe.

Feeding

The couple of days before the ride

During the couple of days before the ride when our horses were on the event place, we aimed at maintaining the feeding program as close as possible to the previous one: same feeds (our concentrate and our hay) that we transported from home; same concentrate quantity fed to the horses; same feeding schedule. The only change was the quantity of hay that was offered ad libitum, during the night before the ride. Even if hay was often provided by the organizer, we preferred to bring hay from home in order to prevent hay refusals or digestive disturbances. On the event place, we provided horses free access to drinking water and salt block. We observed that whereas the average level of intake was 2.6% BW the days before the ride, it went down to 2.3% BW on average one and two days before the race. This decrease was due to a lower consumption of hay (from 2.1 to 1.9% BW) but not to the concentrate intake. We observed high individual variations the day before the ride within three horses diminishing their intake by 30% whereas two did not change and one even increased it by 20%, suggesting different individual management of stressful conditions.

The racing day

Before departure, we offered our horses hay ad libitum but no concentrate. During the ride, one kilogram of the same concentrate as fed usually and hay was presented at each vet gate. Also we offered other types of concentrates in the case that the horses would refuse to eat. As underlined by Crandell (2010), perhaps the single most important key to successful completion of the race is the ability of the horse to eat whenever it has a chance. Water was offered to our horses every 20 minutes on the track and at vet-gates. Although it was a very common practice to supplement horses with electrolytes (Goachet, 2006), our horses were not.

We measured a decrease in feed intake the day of the race that was on average 2.0% BW, mainly due to a decrease in hay intake (from 2.1 pre-ride to 1.4% BW). We also observed important individual variations, with some horses being able to maintain a pre-ride intake while others reduced hay intake to 0.5% BW. Contrary to the other days, the day of the race, horses had a lower time budget for feeding. Also, the required physical effort, the excitement and the fatigue probably contributed to decrease the appetite during the day and the evening. The day of the race, the water intake increased significantly compared to that measured at our animal facilities five days earlier. On average, horses increased their intake by 80% (from 25 to 45 l on average) and depending on the individual this variation varied from 42 to 122%. However 75% of the water was consumed during the vet-gates, within the arrival and the veterinary inspection.

After the race

At the end of the ride and the day after (during the travel back to home), our horses received only hay ad libitum. Interestingly the horses that had the lowest intake the day before the race also had the lowest intake the day of the race and the day after it. When our horses were back home, they had the same feeding program as initially and their level of intake returned to initial values.

How science can serve the field practices

We were guided by the same scientific demands as usual because we were doing experimental trials, even if it was conducted partly in the field. This is why among other things we recorded so many data regarding training, feeding, and shoeing. Honestly we did not think this would ever be useful for other purposes than our research. Today, we realize that our observations allowed generating new knowledge that can be of interest for better managing the endurance horse during training and competition. And we are pleased that science can serve the practitioners in the field.

References

Authie EC, Morillon B, Biau S, Courouce-Malblanc A (2009) Suivi d'entraînement des jeunes chevaux de concours complet d'équitation, à l'entrainement et lors d'épreuves d'aptitude. In: Proc 35th Journées Recherche Equi, Haras Nationaux (ed), France. Pp 169-178.

Barnes A, Kingston J, Beetson S, Kuiper C (2010) Endurance veterinarians detect physiological compromised horses in a 160 km ride. Eq Vet J Suppl 42:6-11.

Benoit P, Barrey E, Regnault JC, Brochet JL (1993) Comparison of the damping effect of different shoeing by the measurement of hoof acceleration. Acta Anatom 146:109-113.

Bergero D, Assenza A, Caola G (2005) Contribution to our knowledge of the physiology and metabolism of endurance horses. Livestock Prod Sci 92:167-176.

Burger D, Dollinger S (1998) Raisons d'élimination, état de santé et carrière sportive des chevaux dans les raids d'endurance en Europe et dans les pays arabes: approche statistique. Pratique Vétérinaire Eq 30:19-25.

Burk AO, Williams CA (2008) Feeding management practices and supplement use in top-level event horses. Comp Exerc Physiol 5:85-93.

Cerchiaro I, Mantovani R, Bailoni L (2004) Indogine sul cavallo da endurance nel Veneto : aspetti gestionali e misere morfologiche (Survey on endurance horse in the Veneto region: management and body measurements). In: Proc Italian Soc Vet Sci, Gorizia, Italy (in Italian, with English abstract).

Clayton HM (1991) Conditioning Sport Horses. Sport Horse Publication, Saskatchewan, Canada.

Cottin F, Metayer N, Goachet AG, Julliand V, Slawinski J, Billat V, Barrey E (2010) Oxygen consumption and gait variables of Arabian endurance horses measured during a field exercise test. Eq Vet J Suppl 42:1-5.

Crandell K (2005) Trends in feeding the American endurance horse. In: Advances in Equine Nutrition III. Pagan J, Geor RJ (eds), Versailles, Kentucky, USA ; Pp 135-138.

Crandell K (2010) Observations and recommendations for feeding the endurance horses. In: Proc Kentucky Eq Res Nutr Conf. Lexington, KY, USA; Pp 132-142.

Danielsen K, Lawrence LM, Siliciano P, Powell D, Thompson K (1995) Effect of diet on weight and plasma variables in endurance exercised horses. Eq Vet J Suppl 18:372-377.

Duren S (1998) Feeding the endurance horse. In: Advances in Equine Nutrition I. Pagan J (ed), Versailles, Kentucky, USA; Pp 351-361.

Gallagher K, Leech J, Stowe H (1992) Protein, energy and dry matter consumption by racing thoroughbreds: a field survey. J Eq Vet Sci 12:43-48.

Geor RJ (2005) Nutritional management of endurance horses. In: Proc 9th Equ Med Surg, Geneva, Switzerland; Pp 38-45.

Glinsky MJ, Smith RM, Spires HR, Davis CL (1976) Measurements of volatile fatty acid production rates in the cecum of the pony. J Anim Sci 42:1465-1470.

Goachet AG (2006) Us et coutumes vs alimentation raisonnée du cheval d'endurance. Congrès de l'AVEF, Versailles, France ; Pp 8.

INRA (1984) Tables des apports alimentaires recommandés pour le cheval. In: Jarrige R, Martin-Rosset W (eds), Le Cheval. Reproduction, Sélection, Alimentation, Exploitation. INRA, Paris ; Pp 645-659.

Julliand V, Ralston S (2006) Ecosystème gastro-intestinal: comment ça marche? Comment ça dysfonctionne? Quelles recommandations en nutrition clinique? Congrès de l'AVEF, Versailles, France. Octobre; Pp 8.

Leclerc JL (2009) L'entraînement du cheval d'endurance: notions fondamentales et évolution. Pratique Vétérinaire Eq 41:7-9.

Liesens L (2009) Endurance: Débuter-Gérer-Gagner. Liesen L (ed), France; Pp 138.

Lopez-Rivero JL, Morales-Lopez JL, Galisteo AM, Aguera E (1991) Muscle fibre type composition in untrained and endurance-trained Andalusian and Arab horses. Eq Vet J 23:91-93.

Marguet C (2009) Etude de prévalence des ulcères gastriques chez le cheval d'endurance. Doctoral thesis Univ Toulouse.

Metayer N, Biau S, Cochet JL, Barrey E (2003) Study of locomotion and conformation in the endurance horse. In: Proc Eur Assoc Anim Prod. Roma, Italy. Abstract H2-10.

Meyer H, Gomba Y, Heilman M (1987) Postprandial renal and recal water and electrolyte excretion in horses in relation to kind of feedstuffs, amount of sodium ingested and exercise. In: Proc Eq Nutr Physiol Symp; Pp 67.

Meyrier S (2003) Les causes d'élimination en épreuves d'endurance équestre: étude rétrospective menée en France en 2001. Doctoral thesis Univ Toulouse.

Munoz A, Cuesta I, Riber C, Gata J, Trigo P, Castejon FM (2006) Trot asymmetry in relation to physical performance and metabolism in equine endurance rides. Eq Vet J Suppl 36:50-54.

Nagy A, Murray JK, Dyson S (2010) Elimination from elite endurance rides in nine countries: a preliminary study. Eq Vet J Suppl 42:637-643.

Nicol CJ (2000) Equine stereotypies. In: Recent Advances in Companion Animal Behavior Problems. Houpt KA (ed), International Veterinary Information Service.

Nieto JE, Snyder JR, Beldomenico P, Aleman M, Kerr JW, Spier SJ (2004) Prevalence of gastric ulcers in endurance horses – a preliminary study. Vet J 167:33-37.

O'Grady S (2008) Basic farriery for the performance horse. Vet Clin North Am Eq Pract 24:203-218.

Parkins T (2009) How to train sport horses: detrimental regimens and exercises. In: Proc Eq Nutr Train Conf, Madrid, Spain; Pp 131-137.

Pélissier C (2009) La ferrure du cheval d'endurance : contraintes et spécificités. Pratique Vétérinaire Eq 41:11-16.

Pietrzak S, Strzelec K (2002) Attempt at a definition of the relationship between conformation and efficiency level in endurance horses. In: Proc Eur Assoc Anim Prod, El Cairo, Egypt. Abstract H3-6.

Prince A, Geor R, Harris P, Hoekstra K, Gardner S, Hudson C, Pagan J (2002) Comparison of the metabolic responses of trained Arabians and Thoroughbreds during high- and low-intensity exercise. Eq Vet J Suppl 34:95-99.

Ralston SL (1988) Nutritional management of horses competing in 160 km races. Cornell Vet 78:53-61.

Robert C, Benamou-Smith A, Leclerc JL (2002) Use of recovery check in long-distance endurance rides. Eq Vet J Suppl 34:106-111.

Valle E, Fusetti L, Bergero D (2009) A survey of feeding practice for show jumping horses in Northern Italy: are scientific new findings being applied? In: Proc Eq Nutr Train Conf, Madrid, Spain; Pp 221-229.

Van Heel MCV, van Weeren PR, Back W (2006). Shoeing sound Warmblood horses with a rolled toe optimises hoof-unrollment and lowers peak loading during breakover. Eq Vet J 38: 258-262.

Warren LK, Lawrence LM, Robert A, O'Connor C, Powell D, Pratt P (2001) The effect of dietary fiber on gastrointestinal fluid volume and the response to dehydration and exercise. In: Proc Eq Nutr Phys Symp. Pp 148-149.

How can we practically manage obese horses and ponies?

Pat Harris
WALTHAM Centre for Pet Nutrition, Freeby lane, Waltham on the Wolds, LEI2 4RT Melton Mowbray, United Kingdom; pat.harris@eu.effem.com

Take home message

The best way to manage an obese horse or pony is to prevent it from becoming obese in the first instance! When managing an animal that has become obese it is obviously key to recognise that it is obese and to put in place a diet and management plan that includes regular monitoring and reviewing. In some individuals initial weight loss may not be accompanied by an obvious change in the externally assessed body condition score.

Key practical management strategies of obese/overweight animals include: (1) promotion of weight loss and improved insulin sensitivity via dietary restriction and, where possible, an increase in physical activity; (2) avoidance of certain feeds that may exacerbate insulin resistance and hyperinsulinemia (feeds rich in non-structural carbohydrates such as grains, high starch containing feeds and 'lush' or stressed pasture forages) and, in some cases (3) treatment with levothyroxine sodium (and potentially other medications – although the efficacy of all of these needs to be proven).

Any weight loss programme needs to be targeted to the individual animal and a process to monitor and review, during and after, the weight loss has been achieved must be established.

Background

Prevalence

A US survey (USDA, 2008) suggested that around 4.5% of their horse population was overweight or obese, but this is likely to be a significant underestimate as it was owner reported. In a prospective US study of 300 randomly selected mature horses, 57 (19%) were classified as obese (Body Condition score [BCS] of 7.5-9.0/9) (Thatcher and colleagues, unpublished data, 2007). In a study of 319 pleasure riding horses in Scotland, 32% were found to be obese (BCS 6 on a 6-point scale) and a further 35% were considered fat (BCS 5/6; Wyse *et al.*, 2008). In a more recent survey, 62% of animals were categorised as being overweight, fat or obese, with a BCS >5/9 and 21% were ≥7/9, despite being in regular work and competing in a national unaffiliated championship show in a variety of equestrian disciplines (Harker *et al.*, 2011).

Health concerns

Chronic obesity may induce a low-grade inflammatory state and equine obesity has been associated with an increased risk of developmental orthopaedic disease (DOD), hyperlipaemia, heat intolerance, insulin insensitivity, increased bone and joint injuries, placental restriction and lowered birth weights (Geor and Harris, 2009). Recently, interest, however, has focused on the apparent increased risk of laminitis in obese ponies (Treiber *et al.*, 2006, 2007; Geor and Harris, 2009; Carter *et al.*, 2009a).

A recently published consensus statement suggested that the majority of equids with equine metabolic syndrome (EMS; Frank *et al.*, 2010) exhibit the following characteristics:

- Generalized obesity or increased adiposity in specific locations, such as the nuchal ligament region (cresty neck).
- Insulin resistance characterized by hyperinsulinaemia or abnormal glycaemic and insulinaemic responses to oral or intravenous glucose and/or insulin challenges.
- A predisposition towards laminitis. Clinical or subclinical laminitis that has developed in the absence of recognized causes such as colic, colitis or retained placenta.

It is important to recognize, however, that not all obese horses are insulin resistant (IR) and that IR can occur in non-obese animals and without raised basal plasma insulin concentrations (Bailey *et al.*, 2008, Carter *et al.*, 2009a,b).

Why obese?

In most cases, the reason why a horse is overweight is because they have stored excess energy/calories as fat, i.e. they have been overfed relative to their activity level. Many horses that spend most of their time in stables with occasional hacks may require no more than maintenance energy intakes, yet many are fed much more than this. Similarly, animals turned out to pasture at certain times of the year may have an intake several times their energy/calorie requirement. It is perhaps surprising that more animals do not become overweight, and this may reflect individual differences in activity levels when out in the field, as well as the ability to convert feed to fat. Certain breeds (e.g. Quarter Horses and Morgans) and types (ponies) are perhaps more prone to obesity and benefit from even closer attention to their diet and exercise.

Native UK pony breeds for example retain strong seasonality with respect to their appetite and under 'feral' conditions tend to gain weight during the summer months when food is abundant before losing it again during the winter. Such cyclical changes may not occur when food intake and quality is maintained during the winter resulting in further weight gain. Recent work has shown differences according to season and initial BCS on weight gain when welsh mountain ponies were fed a fibre based ration *ad libitum* (Dugdale *et al.*, 2011a).

Horses are however, individuals; the amount and type of feed they require to maintain bodyweight plus the desired level of condition and provide the type of ride required therefore depends upon several factors, including:
- age, health and temperament;
- amount and type of work the horse is being asked to carry out;
- environmental conditions;
- body condition required;
- type of ride preferred;
- metabolic and digestive efficiencies.

If a horse is thought to be working hard, as we all recognise, it does not mean that it is actually working hard and even if it is, it does not necessarily mean that more feed or one providing higher energy levels is needed. Hard work does not necessarily mean high energy requirements; similarly, light/medium work does not necessarily mean low energy requirements. Amounts of complementary feed recommended by feed manufacturers can therefore obviously only be a guide.

Management advice

As we learn more about this condition we will be able to provide more detailed and relevant advice but based on our current knowledge this would be the author's advice today.

Key practical management strategies of obese/overweight animals include: (1) promotion of weight loss and improved insulin sensitivity via dietary restriction and, where possible, an increase in physical activity; (2) avoidance of feeds that may exacerbate insulin resistance and hyperinsulinemia (feeds rich in non-structural carbohydrates such as grains, high starch containing feeds and 'lush' or stressed pasture forages); and, in some cases (3) treatment with levothyroxine sodium (and potentially other medications – although the efficacy of all of these needs to be proven, e.g. Tinworth *et al.*, 2011).

Any weight loss programme needs to be targeted to the individual animal but to have a chance to work requires initially:
- Most importantly, the owner/feeder recognising that the animal is overweight, that it needs to lose weight and that this will take time and effort. It is recommended that all veterinarians and owners/ keepers of horses learn to use and apply one system of Body Condition Scoring but appreciate the limitations to such systems (Henneke *et al.*, 1983; Dugdale *et al.*, 2011a,b,c).
- Understanding exactly what is currently being fed (Scoops and haynets should be weighed etc.) Analysing the forage may be required especially in resistant cases (or the decision made to use low energy forage replacers).
- Recognising that potentially up to 40% of the daily dry matter intake can be ingested during just a few hours of turn out (Ince *et al.*, 2011) and up to 1% Body Weight (BW) as Dry Matter (DM) intake within 3hrs (Longland *et al.*, 2011a,b).
- Recognising that some individuals when allowed free access to grass, preserved forage or forage replacers may ingest up to 5% BW of DM per day (Dugdale, 2011a; Longland *et al.*, 2011a,b).

- Being realistic about the amount and type of work the horse actually does and can do.

First stage

Look at the overall diet; if the horse is overweight but still being fed a manufactured diet with plenty of hay or other fibre sources, consider the following feeding strategies. The preferred option will depend on the present and desired bodyweight as well as the individual circumstances.

- Replace the manufactured feed with one providing lower energy, i.e. a high-fibre, low-starch and low-sugar feed, preferably one that has been specifically formulated to help promote weight loss yet maximise the time spent chewing.
- Check the analysis of the current forage; if necessary, change to one providing lower energy levels, such as late seed-cut hay (avoiding high-energy forages such as alfalfa or haylage but also avoid highly indigestible forages). A low-calorie hay replacer may be useful at this stage.
- Restrict access to grass, especially lush pasture, but maintain turn-out by, for example: carefully using appropriate restrictive but not complete exclusion grazing muzzles – appropriately fitted and monitored (Longland *et al.*, 2011b), using strip grazing behind other horses or sheep; mowing and removing clippings; putting a deep layer of woodchips over a small paddock; or using dry lots/ indoor schools. Grazing muzzles must be used with care, should be properly fitted and horses and ponies should be adapted gradually to wearing them. Group and individual behaviour should be monitored closely to observe any potential concerns caused for example by changes to the herd dynamics. Total exclusion muzzles are not advised.

Next stage

The next stage would be to reduce or remove all energy-providing supplementary feed and provide a measured amount of a low energy forage-only diet with minimal intake of grass but the provision of a vitamin- mineral supplement.

- Caution is required when feeding restricted forage intakes on sandy soils for example as potentially there could be an increased risk of sand colic.

Ideally, a combination of one or more of the above measures along with an increase in exercise or activity is recommended. An increase in exercise may be achieved by increasing the number, length or intensity of exercise occasions, or changing the type of formal activity (riding/lunging, etc.), as well as prolonging free activity in the paddock (with a grazing muzzle if required).

Where appropriate, the diet can be made up to near appetite levels by adding low-energy forages, but caution when feeding poorly digested (e.g. high lignin/silicated) forages (especially in significant amounts) which may increase the risk of impaction and gastric ulcers (Luthersson *et al.*, 2009). Consider the use of meal extenders and techniques such as small-holed haynets or haylage nets/double haynets or haylage nets to ensure the horse takes as long as possible to eat the forage provided.

Compound manufactured feeds are formulated to be fed at certain levels. If the amount of feed needed to enable maintenance of a desirable body condition for the horse and preferred type of ride for the rider is less than the manufacturer's recommendation for that workload, an appropriate vitamin and mineral supplement may be necessary. Alternatively, a diet which is less energy-dense should be fed, with appropriate vitamin and mineral fortification.

More severe restrictions

Establishing a programme to promote weight loss may just require restricting grazing, changing the type of forage fed or using a low energy forage replacer and/or reducing the amount or change the type of complementary feed provided as described above – whilst maintaining vitamin and mineral intake to support health.

For some individuals however, more severe restrictions may be required, e.g. as a general guide, for the more obese animals or for those where appropriate changes in the ration as outlined above have not been successful, consider:

- Providing low energy hay (~8 MJ/kg as fed) or forage substitutes initially at ~1.5% of current BW daily (on a Dry-matter intake basis; DMI) with subsequent further reductions if required but the author currently recommends not to decrease to less than 1.0% BW DMI as an absolute minimum unless under appropriate supervision; feeding reduced amounts of fibre may increase the risk for hindgut dysfunction, stereotypical behaviours, gastric ulcers, coprophagy, etc. (Dugdale *et al.*, 2010).
- Straws generally have lower energy contents than good quality horse hays and may be of value to help calorie dilute the ration of some obese animals. But it is important to select clean, carefully harvested straw with minimal cereal heads (also shake thoroughly to remove any loose cereal grains). Straw needs to be introduced into the diet very slowly which helps to reduce the risk of impaction – although this remains a significant risk with certain breeds (eg thoroughbreds) and individuals. The risk of gastric ulceration was also increased in one study when straw was the main forage (Luthersson *et al*, 2009).
- The ration should be divided throughout the day and strategies to prolong feed intake time should be considered, (e.g. nets with multiple small holes).
- It is very important to maintain an appropriate vitamin and mineral intake.
- It is also thought to be important to maintain a good quality protein intake (amino acid profile) to help prevent unwanted muscle loss during more severe weight restriction programmes. The inclusion of exercise in such programmes may be of additional/more value with respect to helping to maintain muscle mass (Dugdale *et al.*, 2010).
- Finally when the management system means that there are animals within sight or hearing that are being fed it may be advisable from a behavioural standpoint to provide a small meal at the same meal times. Ideally ensure any meal fed is sufficiently small in size and low in starch/sugar/energy content.

Individual response

In a recent study, when 12 overweight and obese horses and ponies, were fed 1.25% BW (of fibre based feed ~8 MJ/Kg DM) as DMI over a 16 week controlled weight loss programme, weight loss was unremarkable in four of the animals but quite marked in others (Curtis *et al.*, 2010). This highlights the individual responses to dietary restriction. Even further dietary restriction may be required to achieve significant weight loss in the more 'resistant' animals when increased exercise is not possible. However, currently the author emphasises her recommendation not to reduce fibre intake to < 1.0% BW on a DM intake basis unless under appropriate experienced supervision and management. Much more work is needed in this area.

It is possible that, like other species, as equidae reduce their body weight as a result of restricted energy intake they will reduce their energy expenditure making it difficult to continue to maintain weight loss. The need to reduce the energy intake over the course of the study to maintain BW loss is a common theme in some of the studies reported to date (Van Weyenberg *et al.*, 2008; Gordon *et al.*, 2009). This emphasises the need to individually tailor any weight loss programme and monitor it closely.

Bedding material

Weight management strategies, for obese animals, usually include restricting feed intake and in particular the forage/fibre intake. Especially in the more resistant animals actual feed intake from any source needs to be tightly controlled. Whilst the ingestion of straw from straw beddings may reduce the risk of stereotypical behaviours developing it may result in an increased risk of impaction in certain breeds/individuals and may in fact reduce the effectiveness of any weight management programme due to the amount ingested.

Wood shavings are often advised as an alternative bedding source to help prevent dietary supplementation from this non-controlled non-feed source. Unfortunately, recent work has shown that some individuals may ingest significant amounts of wood shavings when on a weight management programme (Curtis *et al.*, 2011). Up to an estimated 3.5 kg/day was being ingested by one individual in this study without any apparent ill effects. However, impaction remains a risk and further work is required before, scientifically evaluated, recommendations with respect to the optimal bedding for animals within a weight management programme can be given.

Importance of exercise

The importance of exercise with or without a weight loss regimen on body weight and/or level of insulin resistance has been discussed over the years (Freestone *et al.*, 1991, Treiber *et al.*, 2008, Gordon *et al.*, 2009). A very recent study looking at the effect of exercise in obese animals concluded that 'moderate exercise training without concurrent dietary restriction does not mitigate insulin resistance in overweight or obese horses. A more pronounced reduction in adiposity or higher volume or intensity of exercise may be necessary for improvement in insulin sensitivity in such horses' (Carter *et al.*, 2010). Much more work is needed to determine the quantity of physical activity required to positively influence insulin sensitivity in obese animals and to evaluate the effect of weight loss with and without exercise on IR.

In the meantime a program of regular exercise is likely to be beneficial in the management of obese, insulin resistant (but sound) horses and ponies. In the author's experience, weight reduction and subsequent control are improved when dietary restriction is combined with a program of riding or lunging. For those already in work this may involve just increasing the number, length or intensity of the exercise. For those not in work any exercise program needs to be developed in conjunction with the horse/ponies veterinarian and introduced slowly.

Role of medications eg thyroxine

Treatment with levothyroxine sodium (e.g Thyro L®, Lloyd Inc., Shenandoah, IA, USA) has been recommended for horses or ponies with recalcitrant obesity and IR and/or animals with ongoing episodes of laminitis not controlled by more conservative approaches (Frank *et al.*, 2008). Preliminary studies in healthy and EMS horses have demonstrated weight loss and improved insulin sensitivity in *some* animals following a 3-6 month period of levothyroxine sodium treatment. It has been recommended that treated animals should be gradually weaned from the drug when treatment goals have been attained and put on a diet and management program to prevent regain of weight.

More work is needed to evaluate the true efficacy, optimal dose and program for thyroxine and other medications such as metformin (Tinworth *et al.*, 2011).

Time scale

- Do not attempt to make rapid changes to the horse's weight – the absolute maximum amount we would recommend you aim to achieve is 1% body weight per week after the first week, when any weight loss may be due to reduced gut fill. A more realistic (but often still difficult to achieve in the more resistant cases) target is a weekly weight loss of 0.5% (again after the first week) ie 20 kg for a 500 kg horse in ~8-10 weeks.
- Set realistic targets and monitor (under identical conditions) the horse's weight and condition on a regular basis, i.e. every 2-4 weeks. Note that appropriate levels of weight loss may not always be accompanied by significant change in body condition score in the first few months (Dugdale *et al.*, 2010).
- Make all dietary changes gradually and avoid prolonged periods of feed withholding. Abrupt starvation especially in obese ponies, donkeys, and miniature horses (especially pregnant animals) carries the risk for hyperlipemia.
- Develop, and continually update, an appropriate weight maintenance program once the target weight and body condition have been achieved to avoid a return to weight gain. This will include monthly assessment of body weight and condition to ensure that the feeding program is appropriate to the current level of physical activity and other environmental influences on energy requirements (e.g. ambient conditions).

Monitoring

- Calibrated (over the weight range of the horses to be weighed) weighbridges for horses are the most accurate means of monitoring body weight. However, normal fluctuations (up to ~5 kg) may still occur due to feed and water intake, defecation, urination, as well as hydration status (Webb and Weaver, 1979). These can be minimised by measuring at the same time of day/time post feeding, exercise, etc.

- Weigh tapes/formulae may be useful for monitoring purposes – providing they are used by the same person under the same circumstances (position, place of measurement, time post feeding/ exercise, etc.). *Note* that the accuracy of weigh tapes/certain formulae is decreased for adult horses at the extreme ends of the scale, and they may not be applicable for certain classes of horses, including pregnant mares, and thin, fit horses (Gee and Harris, 2005). Formulae/tapes for adults should not be used for foals/growing youngsters (Staniar *et al.*, 2004) and there are now formulae targeted towards specific breed types eg warmbloods (Kienzle and Schramme, 2004).

- Much of a horse's body fat is subcutaneous but it is not spread evenly around the body and therefore tends to accumulate in specific areas. It is these specific and identifiable areas that are examined more closely when using a Body condition scoring (BCS) system. Currently, there are a number of differing systems that can be used to determine condition score (Gee and Harris, 2005). The author currently uses the 1-9 point BCS scale adapted from the original work of Henneke *et al.* (1983) where a score of 1 represents an emaciated animal and 9 an obese animal. Practically an average score is obtained, by dividing the total score by 6 (reflecting the number of body areas examined). Recent work has suggested that in animals with a stable BCS there can be a very close correlation between the BCS using this system and the total soft tissue mass (Dugdale *et al.*, 2011b). In the authors' experience, this system of condition scoring is more able to allow for the changes in body shape often seen for example in older horses, rather than these changes erroneously affecting the score. This helps to reduce the risk that changes within just one part of the body significantly affect the outcome. However, this system was originally developed from work carried out predominantly using Quarter Horse broodmares and is therefore more suited to a lighter breed type of animal, including the Thoroughbred. It has been adapted slightly for the warmblood type of horse (Kienzle and Schramme, 2004).

- Most importantly the amount of total body fat does not increase linearly with increasing body condition score (See Dugdale *et al.*, 2011b). The accuracy for estimating total body fat decreases significantly for animals with a BCS above 6 in the 9 point scale based on the Henneke *et al.* (1983) system. This provides additional support for the exponential relationship described between the

INRA BCS system of 0 to 5 and body fat content in 20 French Sport horses (Martin-Rosset *et al.*, 2008).

- Recently, as least in welsh mountain pony mares, the use of deuterium oxide dilution has been validated for the determination of the % body fat (Dugdale *et al.*, 2011c) and this method has been used in a research setting to monitor weight loss in ponies and horses (Carter *et al.*, 2010; Dugdale *et al.*, 2010) – although it is unlikely to be a routine tool for use in the field.

- Fat ultrasound measurements have been used to provide a guide to the total fat content of a horse but recent work has suggested that this may not be as accurate as previously thought. The various fat depots may behave differently during weight loss or gain and various other parameters including nutritional history, physiological status and even season may influence how fat is distributed within an individual. This means that changes in the depth of a particular fat deposit may not reflect accurately the changes in fat content as measured using deuterium oxide dilution (Dugdale *et al.*, 2010, 2011a,b,c). However, this is a potentially useful monitoring tool and more work is needed to understand how the various depots change under different circumstances.

- The use of bio-impedance analysis (BIA) as a tool to monitor fat loss in the individual animal over time has yet to be proven (and validated against the D_2O dilution method for example), although some interesting preliminary results have been presented (Van der Aa Kuhle *et al.*, 2008).

- Other measurements such as belly girth (with or without correction for height) may prove of more practical value in the future (see Dugdale *et al.*, 2010, 2011a).

What about if they are also prone to laminitis?

Pasture turnout can be a trigger factor for laminitis even in the lean, non-obese animal, which does not have raised basal plasma insulin concentrations. Obesity, however, may increase the risk as does turning out on a pasture with a high non-structural carbohydrate content (simple sugars, fructans, and starch).

Currently based on existing knowledge and scientific reports the author would recommend the following for an obese animal that is also prone to laminitis:

- Base the horse's diet on forage/fibre.
- Especially for horses or ponies that have experienced repeated episodes of laminitis, it is recommended to analyse the forage and to feed a forage with < 10% non-structural carbohydrate (NSC:starch, sugar and fructan) content. Many hays will be higher than this. Soaking grass hay in clean water (>8 °C: winter tap water and ideally around 16 °C: summer tap water) for at least 3hrs may help to reduce the water-soluble carbohydrate (WSC) content (Longland *et al.*, 2010, 2011). However, as the results from soaking are variable it is advisable, if concerned, to ensure the original forage has a low NSC content or feed an appropriate forage replacer.
- Feed a broad-spectrum vitamin and mineral supplement if no or low levels of hard feed are given (or forage is the main component of the diet). Ensure an adequate and balanced intake of magnesium. There is no published scientific evidence, however, to suggest that high levels of magnesium will be protective and reduce the risk of laminitis.
- As the context for these animals is that they are obese – this means that additional energy sources will not be required.
- When the management system means that there are animals within sight or hearing that are being fed it may be advisable from a behavioural standpoint to provide a small meal at the same meal times. Ideally ensure any meal fed is sufficiently small in size and low in starch/sugar/energy content and that it only produces a low/low-moderate insulin response.
- Prevent horses/ponies from having access to grain bins.
- Maintain regular exercise wherever possible.

Advice regarding turn-out:
- Consider zero grazing (whilst providing the horse with suitable forage alternatives) if it is essential that the horse ingests minimal levels of sugar, starch and fructans or you need a strict weight management programme.
- Turn horses out to pasture when fructan/WSC levels are likely to be at the lowest, such as late at night to early morning, removing them from the pasture by mid-morning.
- Do not graze on pastures which have not been properly managed by regular grazing or cutting. Try to maintain a young leafy sward as mature stemmy grasses contain higher levels of stored fructans.

But be aware that herbage yield as well as WSC content per kg dry matter will be important with respect to the overall intake.

- Avoid/restrict turning out in spring (before flower development) and autumn. At any time, consider restricted turnout to pastures during flowering and early seeding.
- Do not allow horses to graze on pastures that have been exposed to low temperatures (e.g. frosts) followed by warm, bright sunny days or those that have been 'stressed' through drought.
- Be aware that ponies have been estimated to be able to eat up to 1% of their bodyweight as dry matter within 3hrs of turnout (Longland *et al.*, 2011a,b).
- Consider maintaining turnout by use of grazing muzzles (Longland *et al.*, 2011b; ensure that horses can obtain sufficient water intake and be aware of possible behavioural issues); strip grazing behind other horses; mowing and removing clippings; putting a deep layer of wood chips over a small paddock or using dry lots/indoor schools, etc.
- Rotate use of paddocks regularly, preferably with other species such as sheep or cattle, to keep the grass levels at an appropriate height to avoid the paddocks becoming 'stressed' through either under or over-grazing.

What about if they are also old?

There is considerable variation in the ageing process in all species and therefore there is no set age at which an individual is automatically considered to be 'geriatric' as opposed to 'aged but healthy'. Some horses remain physically active and healthy well into their twenties and yet others become 'geriatric' by mid teens. These individual differences need to be taken into consideration when determining optimal management and feeding practices. Older healthy horses do not necessarily require any different diet than their younger colleagues – although issues with IR and changes to inflammatory status may occur even in the healthy older animals (See below).

Although the two main clinical situations which are often associated with difficulty in maintaining weight (loss of teeth and abnormal wear patterns; Pituitary pars intemedia dysfunction: PPID) are common in the older horse, in a recent UK survey, ~8% of old horses were reported to be underweight but 10.5% were overweight (Ireland *et al.*,

2011). In Australia, owners of horses and ponies aged ≥15 years (mean 20.5 years) reported that 30% were overweight (BCS 3/5) compared with only 2% which were underweight (BCS < 2/5; McGowan *et al.*, 2010). This suggests that obesity may be as much an issue with older equines as it is in the general horse population.

Peripheral blood mononuclear cells from old horses have increased inflammatory cytokine production compared with those from young animals ('inflamm-aging'). Obese old horses have even greater frequencies of lymphocytes and monocytes producing inflammatory cytokines than do thin old horses and it has been suggested that obesity may play an important role in the apparent age-related dysregulation of inflammatory cytokine production (Adams *et al.*, 2009). Reduction of body weight and body condition in fat old horses significantly reduced the percentage of IFNγ and TNFα positive lymphocytes and monocytes as well as circulating concentrations of TNFα (Adams *et al.*, 2009).

In humans, there is a progressive decrease in insulin sensitivity with age. Recent work (Rapson *et al.*, 2011) reported that there was no difference in the glycemic response to a sweet feed meal in association with age. Healthy aged horses, however, had a greater peak insulin concentration and area under the curve for insulin, than adult horses, regardless of the background diet they had been fed for 5 weeks prior to the meal challenge. These animals were not obese but it could be anticipated that obese older horses may potentially be even more insulin resistant.

Additional nutritional advice

- It would seem even more important to prevent the older horse from being overweight than its younger colleague – but practically this has to be balanced with the often increased difficulties of maintaining body weight of older horses during the winter – especially when they have dental issues. For many older horses, especially if not prone to laminitis, having them in a slightly higher body condition (perhaps 6-7/9) just prior to entering the winter period may be the preferred option. But this does need to be proven.

- However, current advice would be that it might be advisable not to obtain such a body condition score, even if desirable, through the use of meals that promote high insulin responses but to:
  - Consider the use of more digestible forage (i.e. less mature grass hay).
  - Consider including highly digestible fibre sources such as unmollassed sugar beet pulp, soya hulls as a means to increase the energy intake if required without using starch or sugar. The author tends to recommend soaking and throwing away the water even from unmolassed sugar beet pulp to reduce as far as possible the WSC (and fructose) content.
  - If there are no contraindications, consider using oil as an energy source rather than cereal starch – especially for those animals not being exercised (remember to add gradually, balance the overall diet and add additional Vitamin E at 100-150 iu/100 ml of oil). Not more than 1 ml oil/kg BW should be added unless advice has been obtained from a qualified nutritionist or veterinarian.
  - If any cereals, other than oats, are fed make sure they are processed by cooking (e.g. steam flaking, micronising) to make the starch more easily digested, reducing the risk of starch overload.
  - Avoid feeding large grain based meals: restrict meal sizes to < 0.3 kg/100 kg BW of a cereal-based feed. For all horses ensure overall starch intake is < 1 g starch /kg BW per meal.
  - Ideally ensure any meal/forage fed is sufficiently small in size and low in starch/sugar content that it only produces a low (to low-moderate) insulin response.
  - However, again practically it is important to note that for many older horses with poor dentition – access to grazing seems to be the most consistent way to promote a good body condition during the late summer/autumn in preparation for winter.

Conclusion

There is a great deal of exciting and relevant work being undertaken all over the world into this topic. The advice we can give regarding optimal management will therefore be improved and refined as this work is translated into practical application. Until then the above is the author's guide to managing the obese horse and pony but stresses that the above needs to be tailored to the individual animal, owner, and environment.

References

Adams AA, Katepall MP, Kohler K, Reedy SE, Stilz JP, Vick MM Fitzgerald BP, Lawrence LM, Horohov DW (2009) Effect of body condition, bodyweight and adiposity on inflammatory cytokine responses in old horses. Vet Immunol Immunopathology 127:286-294.

Bailey SR, Habsershon-Butcher JL, Ransom KJ, Elliott J, Menzies-Gow NJ (2008) Hypertension and insulin resistance in a mixed-breed population of ponies predisposed to laminitis. Am J Vet Res 69:122-129.

Carter RA, Treiber KH, Geor RJ, Douglass L, Harris P (2009a) Prediction of incipient pasture-associated laminitis from hyperinsulinemia, hyperleptinemia, and generalized and localized obesity in a cohort of ponies. Eq Vet J 41:171-178.

Carter RA, Staniar WB, Cubitt TA, Harris P, Geor RJ (2009a) Apparent adiposity assessed by standardised scoring systems and morphometric measurements in horses and ponies. Vet J 179:204-210.

Carter RA, McCutcheon J, Valle E, Mcilahn EN, Geor RJ (2010) Effects of exercise training on adiposity, insulin sensitivity and plasma hormone and lipid concentrations in overweight or obese insulin-resistant horses Am J Vet Res 71:314-321.

Curtis GC, Barfoot CF, Dugdale AHA, Harris PA, Grove-white D, Argo CMG (2010) Comparison of two, practical weight loss protocols for the management of overweight and obese horses and ponies. In The impact of nutrition on the health and welfare of horses. Ellis AD, Longland AC, Coenen M, Miraglia N (eds) EAAP Publication 128 Wageningen Academic publishers. Pp 237.

Curtis GC, Barfoot CF, Dugdale AHA, Harris PA, McG Argo C (2011) Voluntary ingestion of wood shavings by obese horses under dietary restriction. Br J Nutr (in press).

Dugdale A, Curtis GC, Cripps P, Harris PA, Argo CMcG (2010) Effect of dietary restriction on body condition, composition and welfare of overweight and obese pony mares. Eq Vet J 42:600-610.

Dugdale A, Curtis GC, Cripps P, Harris PA, Argo CMcG (2011a) Effects of season and body condition on appetite, body mass and body. Vet J (in press).

Dugdale AHA, Curtis GC, Harris PA, Mc Argo C (2011b) Assessment of body fat in the pony: Part I. Relationships between the anatomical distribution of adipose tissue, body composition and body condition. Eq Vet J 43(5): 552-561.

Dugdale AHA, Curtis GC, Milne E, Harris PA, Mc Argo C (2011c) Assessment of body fat in the pony: II. Validation of the deuterium oxide dilution technique for the measurement of body fat. Eq Vet J 43(5): 562-570.

Frank N, Geor RJ, Bailey SR, Durham AE, Johnson PJ (2010) Equine metabolic syndrome: ACVIM Consensus Statement. J Vet Int Med 24:467-475.

Frank N, Elliott SB, Boston RC (2008) Effects of long-term oral administration of levothyroxine sodium on glucose dynamics in healthy adult horses. Am J Vet Res 69:76-81.

Freestone JF, Wolfsheimer KJ, Kamerling SG, Church G, Hamra J, Bagwell C (1991) Exercise induced hormonal and metabolic changes in Thoroughbred horses: effects of conditioning and acepromazine. Eq Vet J 23:219-223.

Gee H, Harris PA (2005) Condition scoring and weight estimation: practical tools. In Equine Nutrition for All. Harris PA, Mair TS, Slater JD, Green RE (eds). Proc 1st BEVA and WALTHAM Nutrition symposia Harrogate. Pp 15-24.

Geor RJ, Harris P (2009) Dietary management of obesity and insulin resistance: countering risk for laminitis. Vet Clin North Amer (Eq Pract). Geor RJ (ed) Elsevier Saunders Philadelphia. Pp 51-66.

Gordon ME, Jerina ML, Raub RH, Davison KA, Young JK, Williamson KK (2009) the effects of dietary manipulation and exercise on weight loss and related indices of health in horses. Comp Exerc Physiol 6:33-42.

Harker IJ, Harris PA, Barfoot CF (2011) The body condition score of leisure horses competing at an unaffiliated championship in the UK. J Eq Vet Sci 31:253-254.

Henneke DR, Potter GD, Krieder JL, Yeates (1983) Relationship between condition score, physical measurements and body fat percentage in mares. Eq Vet J 15:371-372.

Ince J, Longland AC, Newbold JC, Harris PA (2011) Changes in proportions of dry matter intakes by ponies with access to pasture and haylage for 3 and 20 hours per day respectively for six weeks. J Eq Vet Sci 31:283.

Ireland JL, Clegg PD, McGowan CM, McKane SA, Pinchbeck GL (2011b) A cross sectional study of geriatric horses in the United Kingdom. Part 2: Health care and disease Eq Vet J 43:37-44.

Kienzle E, Schramme S (2004) Body condition scoring and prediction of bodyweight in adult warm-blooded horses. Pferdeheilkde 20:517-524.

Longland AC, Barfoot C, Harris PA (2010) The effect of water temperature on loss of water-soluble carbohydrates from hay soaked in water for up to 16hrs. In: The impact of nutrition on the health and welfare of horses. Ellis AD, Longland AC, Coenen M, Miraglia N (eds) EAAP Publication 128 Wageningen Academic publishers. Pp 238.

Longland AC, Barfoot C & Harris PA (2011a) Effects of soaking on the water-soluble carbohydrate and crude protein content of hay Vet Rec Published Online First: 7 June 2011 doi.10.1136/vr.d157.

Longland AC, Ince J, Harris PA (2011b) Estimation of pasture intake by ponies from liveweight change during six weeks at pasture. J Eq Vet Sci 31:275-276.

Longland AC, Barfoot C & Harris PA (2011c) The effect of wearing a grazing muzzle vs not wearing a grazing muzzle on pasture dry matter intake by ponies. J Eq Vet Sci 31:282-283.

Luthersson N, Nielsen KH, Harris PA, Parkin TDH (2009) Risk factors associated with equine gastric ulceration syndrome in 201 horses in Denmark. Eq Vet J 41:625-630.

Martin-Rosset W, Vernet J, Dubroeucq H, Arnaud G, Picard A, Vermorel M (2008) Variation of fatness and energy content with body condition score in sport horses and its prediction. In: Nutrition of the exercising horse. Saasamoinene MT, Martin-Rosset W (eds). Eur Assoc Anim Prod 125. Wageningen Academic Publishers, The Netherlands. Pp 167-176.

McGowan TW, Pinchbeck GL, Hodgson DR, McGowan CM (2010) Clinical Disease and mortality in geriatric horses: an Australian Perspective. In: Proc Havemeyer Foundation Equine Geriatric workshop. Pp 23.

Rapson J, Schott II HC, Nielsen BD, McCutchcon LJ, Harris P, Geor RJ (2011) Effects of age and diet on glycemic and insulinemic responses of horses to a concentrate meal. ACVIM (in press).

Staniar WB, Kronfeld DS, Hoffman RM, Wilson JA, Harris PA (2004) Weight prediction from linear measures of growing thoroughbreds. Eq Vet J 36:149-154.

Tinworth KD, Boston RC, Harris PA, Sillence MN, Raidal SL, Noble GK (2011) The effect of oral metformin on insulin sensitivity in insulin resistant ponies. Vet J (in press).

Treiber KH, Kronfeld DS, Geor RJ (2006) Insulin resistance in Equids – Possible role in laminitis. J Nutr 136:2094S-2098S.

Treiber KH, Hess TM, Kronfeld DS, Geor RJ, Boston RC, Harris PA (2007) Insulin resistance and compensation in laminitis-predisposed ponies characterized by the minimal model. Pferdeheilkde 21:91-92.

Treiber KH, Geor RJ, Boston RC, Hess TM, Harris PA, Kronfeld DS (2008) Dietary energy source affects glucose kinetics in trained Arabian geldings at rest and during endurance exercise. J Nutr 138:964-970.

United States Department of Agriculture USDA (2008) NAHMS Equine '98. Part III. Management and Health of Horses (www.aphis.usda.gov/vs/ceah/cahm; accessed Aug 5).

Van der Aa Kuhle K, Cawdell-Smith AJ, Ward LC, Bryden WL (2008) Prediction of equine body composition with bioelectrical impedance spectroscopy. In: Proc Nutr Soc Australia. Adelaide, Australia.

Webb AI, Weaver BMQ (1979) Body composition of the horse. Eq Vet J 11:39-47.

Weyenberg S Van, Hesta M, Buyse J, Janssens GPJ (2008) The effect of weight loss by energy restriction on metabolic profile and glucose tolerance in ponies. JAPAN 92:538-545.

Wyse CA, McNie KA, Tannahil VJ, *et al.* (2008) Prevalence of obesity in riding horses in Scotland. Vet Rec 162:590-591.

Importance of the lactate parameter for performance diagnosis and for the regulation of training in top competition athletics and in recreational sports

Ulrich Hartmann
Institute for Movement and Training Science in Sports II, Faculty of Sport Science, University of Leipzig, Jahnallee 59, 04109 Leipzig, Germany; uhartmann@uni-leipzig.de

General notes on the importance of the lactate parameter in performance diagnosis

In a simplified view, physical capacity during dynamic work or athletic effort lasting for a period of a few minutes can be divided into two ranges:

1. The range of endurance in which energy demands are met entirely through oxygen intake (aerobic range).
2. The range of endurance in which the energy demands for muscle contraction can only be satisfied by additional formation of lactic acid (anaerobic lactic acid range). The resulting increase in the levels of lactate (LA) in the muscle and in the blood (lactate accumulation) leads to metabolic work acidosis. This has an important influence on the performance limit and the resulting state of exhaustion.

Without endurance training, if the maximum capacity during dynamic work for a period of several minutes is measured as the maximum oxygen uptake (VO_2max = 100%), about 70% of this VO_2max is free from net lactate formation and LA build-up (endurance range; [52]). For an individual with extremely highly developed endurance, such as a marathon runner, this range can extend up to 95% of the VO_2max [52].

Between the aerobic and the anaerobic lactic acid ranges of performance, there is a range in which a disproportionately large increase in the blood lactate concentration (LA) with increasing performance marks the start of net lactate formation. This range is usually referred to as the 'transition range' [21] or as the 'aerobic-anaerobic threshold' [54] based on a particular threshold concept (an outline of the various threshold concepts is given in [20]).

It may be accepted as established that if the blood LA concentration curve is recorded during exercise on an ergometer or treadmill with a stepwise or other suitable protocol with increasing effort, the 'limit of endurance' [52, 54] can be determined with reasonable accuracy on the basis of the maximum lactate steady state (MaxLass) during continuous effort, provided that certain basic conditions (durations of steps, duration of intervals, state of nourishment, etc.) are taken into account.

Depending on the course of the test method, this limit lies in the region of the steep increase in the LA concentration [20, 54]; an LA concentration of 4.0 mmol/l may be taken as a reference value for the performance at the 'anaerobic threshold' [52, 54]. It may be assumed that at a constant performance corresponding to an LA level in the region of 4.0 mmol/l, determined with increasing effort and with a step duration of at least five minutes, even prolonged effort still leads on average to a MaxLass in the range from 3.0 to 5.0 mmol/l [20, 21, 54]. The MaxLass can be expected to settle after about 8 to 12 minutes.

If the MaxLass settles in the range 4.0 ± 1.0 mmol/l, the effort can be sustained until the glycogen reserves are exhausted (about 1 to at most 2 hours) [6], provided that there is no delayed further LA increase that forces an earlier termination of the effort [49, 52, 54].

If performance is increased further, the resulting condition of net lactate formation and build-up, associated with the increase in 'lactacidosis', is marked by a more or less steep increase in the LA concentration with time after the first 8 to 12 minutes of effort [49]. The volunteer cannot generally sustain further constant effort for more than 15 minutes [21, 49, 54] if the LA concentration rises above 8 to 12 mmol/l. This is supported by the values found after competitions [18, 38].

It should be mentioned in this context that lactate steady state values higher than 4 mmol/l have been observed in specific exercise studies [2, 40], but these arise partly from the specificity of the sport in question [20].

Determination of the anaerobic threshold by recording the LA performance curve (LPC) in an ergometer test with increasing effort avoids e.g. the risk of a 'vita maxima' effort in the case of a patient or individual with a pathologically reduced performance. Since its reproducibility is generally good, the LPC also provides an objective measure of the lactate-free performance of the volunteer or patient; this can then be used as a measure of endurance.

With the knowledge of the performance at the 'anaerobic threshold', the intensity of endurance training, in both high-level and recreational sports, can be regulated carefully and specifically according to the capacity of the individual, the particular point in the season, and the current training regime.

It has to be mentioned that according to comparative studies, the information provided by MaxLass values based on 'individual anaerobic thresholds' (IATs) or other threshold concepts is no more precise or definite than that obtained by threshold determinations at a fixed LA value of 4 mmol/l [20, 25]. It has been shown that all threshold concepts are subject to certain basic conditions relating to time, and that if these conditions are not taken into account, the interpretation criteria underlying the different threshold definitions cannot be satisfied [20, 21, 23].

A comprehensive overview of the 'transitions' and 'threshold definitions' found in the literature and of the associated methodologies and interpretation procedures can be gained from publications by Heck [20, 24]. It has very recently been proposed [25] that instead of becoming preoccupied with the validity of individual threshold concepts, we should forget about the threshold concepts and abandon the sometimes rather rigid interpretations associated with them.

As will be shown later, however, the optimum and subjectively comfortable training intensity for the development of endurance lies, not in the region of the 'anaerobic threshold' or of the MaxLass, but in a performance range that leads to only a slight elevation of the LA concentration above the resting value (roughly < 2.0 mmol/l). This is only about 70 to 85% of the performance at the threshold. Compliance with this intensity limit in endurance training both by rehabilitation patients and by high-level competition athletes can be checked by LA determination with a direct analyzer during actual training.

General problems with regard to test methods and the interpretation of lactate performance tests in endurance sports

The determination of the 'anaerobic threshold' by ergometric methods as a measure of endurance is subject to certain conditions.

For the LA concentration in the blood to be representative of the LA concentration in the working muscles, the effort in each step must be maintained for a sufficiently long time, certainly for at least 5 minutes [2, 20, 48, 54]. The increase in the effort per step should not exceed a certain value: 30 to 40 watts in bicycle ergometer tests or 0.5 m/s in treadmill tests.

With regard to the duration of the effort step, an up-to-date survey of laboratory test protocols for performance diagnosis [5] shows that even very recently, the basic conditions for test methods as formulated by Mader *et al.* [54] and confirmed by Heck [20] were still being ignored. The shorter the duration of the step, the more the LA distribution leads to a time lag in the LA concentration [21, 22, 24]. Since a short step duration means a shorter LA accumulation time, the LA increase becomes smaller at higher performance levels, and the endurance consequently appears to be better than it really is. It is clear from investigations based on simulation calculations [48] that the interval of about 30 seconds between steps allows partial replenishment of the adenosine triphosphate/creatine phosphate (ATP/CP) pool. Use of the ATP/CP pool is then disproportionately high during the first 30 seconds of the next higher 3-minute effort step, a situation that bears no resemblance to the load conditions occurring in practice. The idea that multi-step tests with short step durations are less time-consuming than other load models is also only an incomplete reflection of reality. Even if this were true, or were to be employed as an argument, it would still be necessary to consider whether it is preferable to spend slightly longer e.g. on tests with longer steps, or to have shorter tests with short steps but less accurate results. Since tests can only be models in any case, we should at least try to make them as realistic as possible. Experience in the regulation of training in recent years has shown that sufficient accuracy can be achieved by the use of heart rates determined in tests with long steps [14, 18, 60].

Another factor that influences the behaviour of the LPC – one that is sometimes overestimated but nevertheless leads to misinterpretations – is the fullness or otherwise of the glycogen store [6]. One type of diet (with a high carbohydrate content) can give the impression of a 'poorer' capacity, while a diet extremely low in carbohydrates leads to the appearance of a 'better' capacity. Effects of this type can be practically eliminated by a normal diet and avoidance of intensive training and competition loads for 1 to 2 days before the performance diagnosis.

It is also regrettable that not enough is known about the relative contributions made by the different types of energy metabolism under the competition loads specific to different sports. Consequently, recommendations regarding improvement targets for training are relatively inexact and vague as far as the energy aspect of performance is concerned. A survey (admittedly not quite up to date) of these relative contributions for many sports is given by Bompa [3].

The literature gives different values for the contributions of the different types of energy metabolism in the various running events [8, 58]. In swimming, the proportions differ according to the particular event, the type of swimmer (short-distance, middle-distance, and long-distance), and the swimmer's condition [62, 72]. For rowing, the proportions have been quantified according to the performance group [17] or the variability during the course of the year [16]. Similar investigations have been conducted for cycling [34], cross-country skiing [62], and canoeing [74], and the results have been summarized in performance structure models. The triathlon events have recently also been the subject of similar studies [60].

Lack of knowledge and/or failure to make use of knowledge about the relationships between the metabolic parameters has led to considerable simplifications in performance diagnosis for endurance sports. Thus, the standard test methods are step tests with relatively short step durations as used in practice, the idea being to test substantially the full spectrum of an athlete's performance on the basis of several successive steps [5]. The 'anaerobic threshold' is determined under these submaximum loads, and is then often (tacitly) equated to the endurance or the 'aerobic capacity'.

The ratio of the maximum performance to the maximum metabolic load, as measured by the maximum post-load lactate value, is used as a source of information about the anaerobic lactic acid component of the energy metabolism or the so-called 'anaerobic capacity'. In training practice itself, efforts are made to determine the maximum performance limit via the criterion of the maximum tolerable LA acidosis [36]. There is a general assumption that quasi-additive combination gives a sufficiently accurate indication of the metabolic capacity. It can be shown with the aid of a few publications that results of this nature are relatively unsatisfactory and vague [48, 51, 52, 54].

A strong correlation can be shown to exist between a submaximum and a maximum capacity in the case of endurance sports that last for 10 minutes or longer. For endurance sports of shorter duration, however, conclusions based on the result of the so-called threshold determination show unsatisfactory agreement with the result of the maximum capacity test, because of a high level of variability (and this situation is aggravated by the different test concepts) [48, 50, 52].

Direct experiments (ergometer testing) alone cannot therefore provide an accurate analysis of the provision of energy during sport-specific (maximum) effort or the answer to the question whether and how utilization of the available metabolic capacities could be optimized or what increases in the proportions of the three metabolic resources would be best for a given competition.

While some authors favour a 'graphic determination' of results in preference to 'software-assisted evaluations' [75], there has been an increase in the use of computer-controlled evaluation methods in recent years [27, 43, 84]. The common aim of the initiators of such methods is to speed up and objectify the presentation of results in lactate performance diagnosis with the aid of computer-assisted evaluation. However, this provides only a partial interpretation [64], if any, of the 'underlying' conditions of the metabolic situation.

A more profound scientifically based interpretation of test results therefore calls for a post-simulation of the experimental observations in a suitably developed simulation model. However, this requires a rather more complex investigation methodology than the simple determination of the performance at 4 mmol/l.

The possibilities offered by a computer-assisted post-simulation can be seen from a number of recent publications [48, 50, 51, 52]. The authors demonstrate how much the maximum aerobic and anaerobic work capacities affect one another when the duration of the event is taken into account and according to the condition of the individual, and they show how slightly varied and sometimes different metabolic patterns, and the consequences associated with them, can lead to similar performances. The resulting interpretations go far beyond the current range of routine performance diagnosis, which is dominated by a preoccupation with lactate. Though these interpretation models result from what appears to be a purely theoretical approach, they nevertheless lead, if used appropriately, to an explanation of the possible variability of the metabolic situations in the realization of a performance [48]. Another effect of the computer-assisted interpretation method is that subjective influences due to the observer are pushed largely into the background, and this leaves room for a much more objective assessment of a given metabolic situation.

Fundamental studies on questions of performance diagnosis have existed for some time for various sports in which endurance plays a major role. The importance of LA performance diagnosis in connection with running events [8, 58, 59, 68], canoeing [74], cycling [31, 34, 65], rowing [18, 19], swimming [62, 72], the triathlon [7, 60], and a number of other endurance sports [62, 66] is undisputed, and this has now become a part of routine management in these sports.

Lactate as a diagnostic parameter in team sports

There have also been many studies on the use of LA in performance diagnosis and training management for team sports, and particularly for football [9, 10, 11, 13, 28, 44, 45, 56, 57, 73, 81].

There is as yet no accurate description and quantification of the basic conditions with regard to energy for individual team sports. Estimates of sprinting capacity and endurance have been published for football [44, 81], but this has not yet led to definite clarification of the relative contributions made by the various energy supply mechanisms.

In the application of lactate performance diagnosis, it must be assumed that running capacities similar to those found in treadmill tests e.g. for excellent middle-distance and long-distance runners are not appropriate objectives for team sports (see above; [9, 10]). It seems unwise to base training plans for team sports directly on findings relating to the improvement of metabolic capacity in endurance-oriented sports [11].

Knowledge of a reference or threshold value is certainly necessary for the general assessment of individual running performance several times per year for team sports [10, 37, 44]. According to the information in the literature [56], which tends to be rather general, the main objective of the battery of tests consisting of several individual investigations should be to provide the athletes with LA-oriented individual estimates of their running intensities and to provide the trainer with an indication of the running speeds in the various load ranges [56]. Individual adjustment of training or training groups based on different physical endurance performances [13, 81] is a practice that is encouraged and pursued on the whole.

Lactate as a parameter of intensity regulation in endurance sports

A search through the literature on training science reveals that decisive qualitative characteristics for performance development are ascribed to certain intensity ranges in endurance training [15, 82, 83]. Many general recommendations are made on this basis with regard to the intensities required in endurance sports.

In connection with training for middle-distance (1000 m) running events, one source mentions that for improved aerobic capacity it is necessary to 'work in the region of the aerobic/anaerobic threshold' [29]. It is also stated that '¼ a high quantity/low intensity training pattern to improve aerobic capacity' is considered to be 'a way of killing time and a pointless pursuit of km ¼' [29]. These and other opinions [36] have led to training plans centred on the 'attainment of high hyperacidity' [70] for the development of capacity over 400 m and for middle distances.

With the aid of a classification, Föhrenbach [9] has quantified the training methods for running events, and has shown the metabolic ranges in which middle-distance and long-distance female athletes trained according to the time of year. For 800 m runners, the more intense load units (LA >4 mmol/l) accounted for between 20 and 35% of all training, while the remaining 80 to 65% of running training took place in LA ranges up to 4 mmol/l. The corresponding ranges for 3000 m runners were estimated to be about 0 to 15% and 100 to 85%.

Another questionnaire [9] revealed that the LA values during the training of female marathon runners were 'mainly under the lowest possible lactic acid load of around 1.0 mmol/l ¾ corresponding to 80-86% of the test running speed at 2.5 mmol/l ¼'.

Vassiliadis *et al.* [79] have also classified the training methods of middle-distance runners, and have shown that about 85% of all training loads corresponded to LA values in the range from the resting LA up to 2.5 mmol/l. About 10% of training took place at LA levels between 2.5 and 4 or 6 mmol/l, and the remaining 5% of all loads, including all competitions, are distributed over intensities above 4 or 6 mmol/l (oral communication).

Neumann *et al.* (1993) report that 60% of training for the triathlon in the case of high-ranking athletes, and 80% in the very highest ranks, takes place in a metabolic range expected to correspond to an LA level of less than 2.0 mmol/l.

Suggestions that training for cross-country skiing should take place at an LA level of about 6 mmol/l have proved to be incorrect [45]. There has been a report of basic endurance training for a long time in the LA range from 2.0 to 3.0 mmol/l [55], but it is unlikely that this would be feasible with large amounts of training.

Similar assumptions have been made with regard to the effectiveness of endurance training in rowing; thus, loads are considered to have 'a stabilizing effect on aerobic capacity' only if they 'produce a LA value of between 2.5 and 3.0 mmol/l' [12]. It is also conjectured that loads in this range 'account for the majority of rowing training and allow rowing times of about 2.0 to 2.5 hours per training unit' [12].

Other literature sources indicate that 'stabilization of aerobic capacity' goes hand in hand with 'LA values around 2.5 to 3.5 mmol/l' [77], that 'the main loads' can be expected in the LA range between 3.5 and 6.0 mmol/l [61], and that endurance training is effective only if it takes place at LA values in the region of 4 mmol/l [12]. Other studies report that relatively low LA values were found after long-distance loads, despite the fact that it had been intended to reach higher values [47, 77].

The training aids catalogue drawn up in the former GDR (German Democratic Republic, East Germany) for endurance sports and tailored to the methodological requirements of rowing also suggests, through the concept 'GAE = Grundlagenausdauer entwickelnd' (basic endurance developing) (LA 3-4 mmol/l [1]) or 'development range' [39], that only training within this range can be effective.

It is reported elsewhere that 'loads in the region of the aerobic threshold (LA formation approx. 2 mmol/l) and below ¼ have progressively less effect on the development of aerobic capacity' [12]. A similar message can also be drawn from the training classifications of the former GDR, according to which the LA range below 2 mmol/l is of little or no importance [1, 39].

In the case of rowing, the intensity values deduced from or recommended in the literature are in conflict with many results from field studies [18, 19]. Thus, it has been shown that for extensive endurance training, long training times at rowing loads leading to LA values in the region of 1.5 mmol/l for up to 75% of total training and 90% of water training may be regarded as correct and important for the improvement and maintenance of performance [18]. There is neither any physiological basis nor any practical evidence to support the idea that training mainly in the LA range from 3 to 4 mmol/l, or at even higher intensities, is more effective.

According to Reiß *et al.* [67], it has been found at the highest levels of athletics that only work ranges above the existing limit are effective. It is assumed that the aerobic-anaerobic transition range can be improved both by exceeding the usual load duration and by increasing the load intensity while keeping the duration constant. No scientific evidence is given in support of these claims.

It appears from our own investigations [18, 19] and from practical [9, 46, 69, 79] and theoretical studies by other authors [25, 26] that the majority of the literature data do not correspond to the conditions found in practice.

Similar results were obtained by Mader [48, 49, 51, 52] on the basis of simulation calculations for middle-distance and long-distance running.

From the arguments that can be gleaned from the publications (see above), it is possible to explain and to understand why some of the intensity recommendations in the literature are not feasible either in practice or in theory.

These observations are not intended to suggest that the intensity range between 2 and 6 mmol/l is not important. However, the percentages of training that actually take place in this intensity range fall far short of the values and recommendations found in the literature (see above).

The desperation that led to the erroneous intensity ideas revealed in the literature springs from the general problem of an insufficiency or a total lack of objective training data based on the actual metabolic demands made by the particular (endurance) sport. The intensity recommendations adopted in the literature of sports medicine and training science certainly sometimes provide definite guidance on training loads, but no theoretical or practical checking has taken place.

Heck *et al.* [25] came to the same conclusion. These authors believe that basic empirical investigations must be conducted in many branches of sport in order to establish the amounts of training and the lactate-based intensities that lead to the best results [25].

Ulrich Hartmann

Limitations of the use of lactate for the regulation of training in endurance sports

As has been shown above, the use of the LA parameter in the regulation of training sometimes leads to the impression that effective training must always be associated with the attainment of certain lactate ranges in training or with the achievement of certain LA values in relation to a corresponding load.

With a number of sports as example, it has been possible to show that the majority of training takes place in a range that is substantially free from LA accumulation [9, 14, 18, 60]. Our own investigations have revealed that in long-distance rowing, an oxygen uptake (VO_2) corresponding to about 50 to 60% of the VO_2max of about 6 l/min can be expected without causing the LA to rise above 1.5 to 2.0 mmol/min. Sporadic studies in connection with middle-distance and long-distance track-and-field events have led to a similar result.

On the assumption of slightly higher load intensities in accordance with the literature recommendations and simultaneous adherence to the indicated amounts of training, it would not be possible to reconcile the caloric demand for training, or the corresponding fraction of the glycogen consumption, with the available regeneration times. In connection with training for endurance sports of medium duration (duration of load >3 minutes), it is sometimes argued that by shifting amount-oriented training to more intensity-oriented loads it is possible to keep the total effort unchanged or nearly so; however, this is questionable on energy grounds alone.

Simulation calculations by Mader [49, 50] based on middle-distance and long-distance running events show that depending on the athlete's condition, it may be advisable to limit O_2 uptake values in endurance training to about 50 to 60% of the VO_2max, or not more than 30 to 40% with a corresponding contribution from the burning of carbohydrates.

It must therefore be concluded that training stimuli or training adjustments cannot be decided purely on the basis of adherence to or attainment of specified LA values during training. The metabolic particulars of the individual athlete are also important factors that must be taken into account. General recommendations based exclusively on LA values lead to a generalization of training loads and a failure to consider the high loads to which the oxidative system is actually subjected.

Importance of lactate studies in recreational sports

In view of the foregoing, it could be surmised that a very sceptical attitude should be taken towards LA studies in recreational sports, and that the application of such studies seems very dubious. It may be assumed that endurance training for recreational sports will consist of 2 to 4 units per week with not more than 60 minutes of effort per training unit. On this basis it should be possible to expect endurance corresponding to a LA value of 4 mmol/l at a VO_2 of about 50 to 70%. LA accumulation with loads in excess of 4 mmol/l can accordingly be expected to begin in this range (see above). Training intensities above this limit are certainly feasible for short periods, but it is unlikely that they will constitute ideal training or that they will improve the endurance to the desired degree.

Field studies in recreational sports have shown that LA values of up to 12 mmol/l [80] are by no means unusual in leisure joggers. Since the intervals between training units in leisure and recreational sports are relatively long (about 48 to 72 hours), it may be assumed that recovery is practically complete, based on the glycogen reserves [6]. If we also consider that somewhat more intensive training (LA values in the region of 4 mmol/l) leads to subjectively more pleasant training as a result of sympathetic activation, it becomes possible to understand the predominance of the tendency, in recreational and leisure sports, towards more intensive loads associated with correspondingly higher LA values [4]. A more detailed examination would be necessary before we could conclude on this basis that the LA range around 2 mmol/l is the lowest intensity for the improvement of endurance in recreational and leisure sports [4]. As other authors have demonstrated [32, 33, 41, 42, 80], however, facilities for LA determinations with a direct analyzer using capillary blood from an ear lobe or from a finger tip can assist with the regulation of subjectively grossly incorrect estimates of training loads, and so help to avoid excessive physical strain. If these determinations are used in conjunction with individual monitoring of the heart rate [30, 71] or of a measure of running intensity [41] for a recreational athlete trained to a relatively good level of endurance, the result is a fairly close approach to what is regarded as practically ideal regulation of training in recreational sports.

Also in the area of recreational and leisure sports, or perhaps particularly in this area, it must be assumed that the manifest objective should not be the attainment of certain LA concentrations during athletic effort, whatever its nature, but that the emphasis should be on moving away from the idea of specified or even higher load intensities.

Conclusions

The purpose of the arguments presented was to point out the problems associated with performance diagnosis and the regulation of training based on the lactate parameter in endurance sports, but also to indicate the possibilities that it has to offer, which will call for a more discriminating approach in the future.

In view of the large body of basic findings, the importance of lactate for performance diagnosis cannot be denied, despite difficulties of interpretation due to the relationships reported above. This importance is shown both by the potential for practical use in routine performance diagnosis and by the discoveries made in recent years through field studies concerning the possibilities for the regulation of training in individual branches of sport. The idea of abandoning the use of the lactate parameter in sports medicine and in practical training science seems unthinkable.

To summarize, it must be concluded that lactate is a parameter of the anaerobic lactic acid energy metabolism, and that its use allows only an indirect and incomplete estimate or interpretation of a particular metabolic situation, always with a bias towards the conditions of one particular sport discipline. The current predominantly clinical approach to lactate ignores many of the recent findings, and sometimes leads to the propagation of erroneous ideas. For this reason, there is a pressing need to take into account the load structure and training practice in the individual sport disciplines.

Interpretation aids for better identification of given metabolic conditions through the use of computer-assisted methods will become increasingly important in the future, at least at the higher levels of competitive sports.

References

1. Altenburg D, Schmidt HP (1991) Rahmentrainingsempfehlungen des deutschen Ruderverbandes für Junioren 1991/92. Handreichungen für Trainer. Ratzeburg: Eigenverlag Deutscher Ruderverband.

2. Benecke R, Boldt F, Meller W, Behn C (1991) Das maximale Laktat-Steady-State im Eisschnellauf. In: Bernett P, Jeschke D (eds). Sport und Medizin – Pro und Contra; München; Zuckschwerdt; Pp 799-767.

3. Bompa T (1990) Theory and methodology of training: the key to athletic performance. Dubuque, Iowa: Kendall.

4. Buskies W, Kläger G, Riedle H (1992) Möglichkeiten zur Steuerung der Belastungsintensität für ein breitensportlich orientiertes Laufausdauertraining. Dtsch Zts Sportmed 42: 248-260.

5. Clasing D (1994) Leistungsdiagnostik – (sportartspezifische) Tests im Labor. In: Clasing D, Weicker H, Böning D (eds). Stellenwert der Laktatbestimmung in der Leistungsdiagnostik. Stuttgart-Jena-New-York: Fischer; Pp 221 227.

6. Costill DL, Sparks R, Gregor R, Turner G (1971) Muscle glycogen utilization during exhaustive running. J Appl Physiol 31:353-356.

7. Föhrenbach R (1990) Leistungsdiagnostik, Trainingsanalyse und -steuerung im Triathlon. Leistungssport 20:35-40.

8. Föhrenbach R (1986) Leistungsdiagnostik, Trainingsanalyse und -steuerung bei Läuferinnen und Läufern verschiedener Laufdisziplinen. Konstanz: Hartung-Gorre.

9. Föhrenbach R, Buschmann J, Liesen H, Hollmann W, Mader A (1986) Schnelligkeit und Ausdauer bei Fußballspielern unterschiedlicher Spielklassen. Schweiz Zts Sportmed 34:113-119.

10. Föhrenbach R, Buschmann J, Mader A, Hollmann W (1993) Speed and endurance in soccer: A comparison of professional and amateur players. Science and Football 7:24-31.

11. Föhrenbach R, Frick U, Göbel M, Nagel P, Stutz R, Schmidtbleicher D, Böhmer D (1991) Dauerlauf- versus Intervalltraining. Dtsch Zts Sportmed 42:136-146.

12. Fritsch W (1981) Zur Entwicklung der speziellen Ausdauer im Rudern. In: Deutscher Sportbund (eds). Informationen zum Training: Rudern (Beiheft zu Leistungssport, Heft 26). Frankfurt: Pp 4-32.

13. Gerisch G, Weber K (1992) Diagnostik der Ausdauer und Schnelligkeit im Leistungsfußball. Fußballtraining 10 (8):32-38 and 10 (9):32-38.

14. Grabow V (1994) Zur Aussagefähigkeit standardisierter Ergometrie- und Feldbelastungen für die Leistungssteuerung in der Sportart Rudern. In: Brack R, Hohmann A, Wieland H (eds). Trainingssteuerung: Konzeptionelle und trainingsmethodische Aspekte, Stuttgart, Germany; Pp 127-132.

15. Grosser M, Brüggemann P, Zintl F (1986) Leistungssteuerung in Training und Wettkampf. München-Wien-Zürich: BLV.

16. Hartmann U, Mader A, Hollmann W (1988) Die Beziehung zwischen Laktat, Sauerstoffaufnahme und Leistung in einem zweistufigen Ruderergometertest bei Ruderern unterschiedlicher Leistungsfähigkeit. In: Steinacker JM (ed). Rudern: Sportmedizinische und sportwissenschaftliche Aspekte. Berlin-Heidelberg-London-Paris-New York-Tokyo: Springer; Pp 110-117.

17. Hartmann U, Mader A, Hollmann W (1987) Querschnittsuntersuchungen an Leistungsruderern mit einem zweistufigen Test auf dem Gjessing-Ruderergometer. In: Rieckert H (ed). Sportmedizin – Kursbestimmung. Berlin-Heidelberg-New York-London-Paris-Tokyo: Springer; Pp 537-544.

18. Hartmann U, Mader A, Petersmann G, Grabow V, Hollmann W (1989) Verhalten von Herzfrequenz und Laktat während ruderspezifischer Trainingsmethoden. Untersuchungen bei A- und B-Kaderruderern und deren Interpretation für die Trainingssteuerung. Dtsch Zts Sportmed 40:200-212.

19. Hartmann U, Mader A, Grabow V, Wittkamp O, Komanns B (1993) Verteilung von Trainingsintensitäten weiblicher Hochleistungsruderer in der Trainingspraxis. In: Martin D, Weigelt S (eds). Trainingswissenschaft. Selbstverständnis und Forschungsansätze; Sankt Augustin: Academia 1:233-243.

20. Heck H (1992) Laktat in der Sportmedizin. Schorndorf: Hofmann.

21. Heck H, Hess G, Mader A (1985) Vergleichende Untersuchungen zu verschiedenen Laktat-Schwellenkonzepten. Dtsch Z Sportmed 36:19-25.

22. Heck H, Liesen H, Mader A, Hollmann W (1981) Der Einfluß der Stufendauer und der Pausendauer bei Laufbanduntersuchungen auf die Sauerstoffaufnahme und das Laktatverhalten. In: Kindermann W, Hort W (eds). Sportmedizin für Breiten- und Leistungssport. Gräfeling: Demeter; Pp 245-253.

23. Heck H, Mader A, Hess G, Mücke S, Müller R, Hollmann W (1985) Justification of the 4 mmol/l lactate threshold. Int J Sports Med 6:117-130.

24. Heck H, Mader A, Müller R, Hollmann W (1986) Laktatschwellen und Trainingssteuerung. Dtsch Zts Sportmed 37:72-78.

25. Heck H, Rosskopf P (1993) Die Laktat-Leistungsdiagnostik – valider ohne Schwellenkonzepte. TW Sport & Medizin 5:344-352.

26. Heck H, Roßkopf P (1994) Grundlagen verschiedener Laktatschwellenkonzepte und ihre Bedeutung für die Trainingssteuerung. In: Clasing D, Weicker H, Böning D (eds). Stellenwert der Laktatbestimmung in der Leistungsdiagnostik. Stuttgart-Jena-New York: Fischer; Pp 111-131.

27. Hille CT, Geiger LV (1993) Mathematische Beschreibung der Laktatkinetik beim Stufentest und Umsetzung in eine datenbankorientierte Analysen-Software. Leistungssport 25:46-51.

28. Hillmann W, Liesen H, Budinger H, Hollmann W (1983) Untersuchungen zur anaerob-laktaziden Belastung im Hallenhockeytraining und -spiel. In: Heck H, Hollmann W, Liesen H, Rost R (eds). Sport: Leistung und Gesundheit. Köln: Dt. Sportärztekongreß; Pp 583-590.

29. Hirsch L (1977) Trainingsformen zur Verbesserung der aeroben Kapazität. In: Deutscher Sportbund (ed). Informationen zum Training: Ausdauertraining, Stoffwechselgrundlagen und Steuerungansätze (Supplement to Leistungssport, 9). Frankfurt; Pp 93-103.

30. Hollmann W, Mader A, Liesen H, Heck H, Rost R (986) Die aerobe Leistungsfähigkeit. Spektrum der Wissenschaft 9:48-58.

31. Hörner J, Buhl H, Licht G (1985) Belastungs- und Leistungssteigerung im 4000-M-Einzelverfolgungsfahren durch Erhöhung des Trainingsumfangs im aerob-anaeroben Übergangsbereich in Verbindung mit einer veränderten zyklischen Gestaltung des Trainings im Grundlagenausdauerbereich II und im wettkampfspezifischen Bereich. Forschungsbericht FKS, Leipzig.

32. Jablonski D, Liesen H, Kraus J, Mödder H (1985) Intensitätssteuerung und Leistungsbeurteilung beim Jogging. Fortschritte der Medizin 103:27-32.

33. Jablonski D, Liesen H, Hollmann W (1987) Untersuchungen zur Entwicklung eines Trainingsgefühls zur Intensitätssteuerung des Dauerlauftrainings bei älteren Frauen und Männern. In: Rieckert H (ed). Sportmedizin – Kursbestimmung. Berlin-Heidelberg-New York-London-Paris-Tokyo: Springer; Pp 34-38.

34. Kettmann S (1983) Erfahrungen und Erkenntnisse bei der zielorientierten Auswertung leistungsdiagnostischer Resultate im Straßenradsport. Theorie und Praxis Leistungssport 21:49-60.

35. Kindermann W (1977) Anaerobe Energiebereitstellung im Hochleistungssport. Schorndorf: Hofmann.

36. Kindermann W (1984) Grundlagen der anaeroben Leistungsdiagnostik. Schweiz Zts Sportmed 32:69-74.

37. Kindermann W, Gabriel H, Coen B, Urhausen A (1993) Sportmedizinische Leistungsdiagnostik im Fußball. Dtsch Z Sportmed 44:232-244.

38. Kindermann W, Haralambie G, Kock J, Keul J (1973) Säure-Basen-Haushalt und Laktatspiegel im arteriellen Blut bei Ruderern nach olympischen Wettkämpfen. Med Welt 24:1176-1178.

39. Körner T, Schwanitz P (1987) Rudern. Berlin: Sportverlag.

40. Krüger J, Schnettler S, Heck H, Hollmann W (1990) Relationship between rectangular triangular inreasing work load and maximal lactate steady state on

the crank ergometer. Sports, Medicine and Health; In: Hermans GPH, Mosterd WL (eds); Amsterdam: Excerpta Medica; Pp 685-690.

41. Lagerström D, Graf J (1986) Die richtige Trainingspulsfrequenz beim Ausdauersport. Herz, Sport und Gesundheit 3:21-24.

42. Lagerström D (1994) Grundlagen der Sporttherapie bei koronarer Herzkrankheit. Köln: Echo-Verlag.

43. Leitner H, Hofmann P, Leitner K (1992) Software zur Auswertung von Herzfrequenz- und Laktatwerten in der Leistungsdiagnostik. Österr J Sportmed 22:115-118.

44. Liesen H (1983) Schnelligkeitsausdauertraining im Fußball aus sportmedizinischer Sicht. Fußballtraining 1:27-31.

45. Liesen H, Hillmann W, Kleiter K, Budinger H (1985) Neue Wege zu besserem Hockeytraining. Allgemeine sportmedizinische Aspekte. Deutsche Hockeyzeitung, Teil III-VI:8-15.

46. Liesen H, Ludemann E, Schmengler D, Föhrenbach R, Mader A (1985) Trainingssteuerung im Hochleistungssport: Einige Aspekte und Beispiele. Dtsch Z Sportmed 36:8-18.

47. Lormes W, Michalsky R, Grünert-Fuchs M, Steinacker JM (1988) Belastung und Beanspruchungsempfinden im Rudern. In: Steinacker JM (ed). Rudern: Sportmedizinische und sportwissenschaftliche Aspekte. Berlin-Heidelberg-London-Paris-New York-Tokyo: Springer; Pp 332-336.

48. Mader A (1994) Aussagekraft der Laktatleistungskurve in Kombination mit anaeroben Tests zur Bestimmung der Stoffwechselkapazität. In: Clasing D, Weicker H, Böning D (eds). Stellenwert der Laktatbestimmung in der Leistungsdiagnostik. Stuttgart-Jena-New York: Fischer; Pp 133-152.

49. Mader A (1994) Die Komponenten der Stoffwechselleistung in den leichtathletischen Ausdauerdisziplinen – Bedeutung für die Wettkampfleistung und Möglichkeiten zu ihrer Bestimmung. In: Tschiene P (ed). Neue Tendenzen im Ausdauertraining. Informationen zum Leistungssport, Band 12 (Bundesausschuss Leistungssport). Frankfurt am Main, Germany; Eigenverlag; Pp 127-216.

50. Mader A (1991) Evaluation of the endurance performance of marathon runners and theoretical analysis of test results. J Sports Med Phys Fitness 31:1-19.

51. Mader A, Hartmann U, Hollmann W (1988) Der Einfluß der Ausdauer auf die 6 minütige maximale anaerobe und aerobe Arbeitskapazität eines Eliteruderers. In: Steinacker JM (ed). Rudern: Sportmedizinische und sportwissenschaftliche Aspekte. Berlin-Heidelberg-London-Paris-New York-Tokyo: Springer; Pp 62-78.

52. Mader A, Heck H (1991) Möglichkeiten und Aufgaben in der Forschung und Praxis der Humanleistungsphysiologie. Spect Sportwissen 3:5-54.

53. Mader A, Heck H (1986) A theory of the metabolic origin of anaerobic threshold. Int J Sports Med 7 (Supplement 1):45-65.

54. Mader A, Hollmann W (1977) Zur Bedeutung der Stoffwechselleistungsfähigkeit des Eliteruderers in Training und Wettkampf. In: Deutscher Sportbund (ed). Informationen zum Training: Ausdauertraining, Stoffwechselgrundlagen und Steuerungsansätze (Supplement to Leistungssport 9). Frankfurt; Pp 8-62.

55. Martin D (1985) Probleme und Fragestellungen der Trainingssteuerung bei Ausdauerentwicklung. Leistungssport 15:7-14.

56. Mücke S, Liesen H (1993) Ausdauerleistungsdiagnostik im Fußball. In: Tittel K, Arndt KH, Hollmann W (eds). Sportmedizin gestern-heute-morgen. Leipzig-Berlin-Heidelberg: Barth; Pp 293-297.

57. Mücke S, Schneider P, Peters B, Liesen H (1991) Trainingssteuernde Maßnahmen bei jugendlichen Hockeyspielerinnen während einer Hallensaison. Leistungssport 21:40-42.

58. Neumann G (1990) Leistungsstruktur in den Ausdauersportarten aus sportmedizinischer Sicht. Leistungssport 20:14-20.

59. Neumann G (1991) Zur Leistungsstruktur der Kurz- und Mittelzeit-Ausdauersportarten aus sportmedizinischer Sicht. Leistungssport 21:29-32.

60. Neumann G, Pfützner A, Hottenrott K (1993) Alles unter Kontrolle; Ausdauertraining. Aachen: Meyer und Meyer.

61. Nolte V (1986) Trainingssteuerung – Voraussetzungen, Anwendung, Grenzen. Leistungssport 16:39-43.

62. Olbrecht J (1989) Metabolische Beanspruchung bei Wettkampfschwimmern unterschiedlicher Leistungsfähigkeit. Doctoral thesis, Univ. Cologne.

63. Ostrowski G (1983) Zur Erhöhung der Wirksamkeit der zentralen Leistungsdiagnostik für die Steuerung und Regelung des Trainings im Skilanglauf. Theorie und Praxis. Leistungssport 21:81-89.

64. Pansold B, Roth W, Zinner J, Hasart E, Gabriel B (1982) Die Laktat-Leistungskurve – ein Grundprinzip sportmedizinischer Leistungsdiagnostik. Med Sport 22:107-112.

65. Petermann A, Kettmann S, Scharschmidt F (1988) Erarbeitung theoretischer Grundpositionen zum 100 km-Mannschaftszeitfahren und ihre praktische Erprobung als Alternativprogramm sowie bei der Olympiavorbereitung – Beitrag zur Leistungssteigerung im 100 km-Mannschaftszeitfahren. Forschungsbericht FKS. Leipzig.

66. Reinke C, Bauer P, Jünger S (1988) Analyse der physiologischen Struktur der 5000 M-Leistung der Männer. Forschungsbericht FKS. Leipzig.

67. Reiß M, Pfeiffer U (1991) Leistungsreserven im Ausdauertraining. Berlin: Sportverlag.

68. Reiß M, Löffler P, Schmidt P, Schön R (1993) Schlüsselprobleme des langfristigen Leistungsaufbaus. Leistungssport 23:12-16.

69. Roth W, Hasart E, Wolf WV, Pansold B (1993) Untersuchungen zur Dynamik der Energiebereitstellung während maximaler Mittelzeitausdauerbelastung. Med Sport 23:107-114.

70. Schmidt P (1977) Trainingsformen zur Erzielung einer hohen Übersäuerung. In: Deutscher Sportbund (ed). Informationen zum Training: Ausdauertraining, Stoffwechselgrundlagen und Steuerungsansätze (Supplement to Leistungssport 9). Frankfurt:104-111.

71. Schmith G, Israel S (1983) Herzschlagfrequenz beim gesundheitsorientierten Ausdauertraining: 170 – ½ Lebensalter (Jahre) ± 10 Jahre. Med. u. Sport 23:158-161.

72. Stafenk W, Appelt D, Hüttner C, Leobold H, Schwalbe W, Chmelik D, Knofe R (1985) Zur weiteren Aufhellung der Leistungsstruktur und Präzisierung der Trainingsstruktur insbesondere unter Beachtung von Fähigkeitskomplexen in Einheit mit der sportlichen Technik (Teil I). Forschungsbericht, FKS. Leipzig.

73. Tritschoks HJ, Gerisch G, Ferrauti A, Weber K (1993) Metabolische Beanspruchung im Hallenfußball. In: Tittel K, Arndt KH, Hollmann W (eds). Sportmedizin gestern-heute-morgen. Leipzig-Berlin-Heidelberg: Barth; Pp 166-169.

74. Ueberschär I, Heinz M, Rühl H (1990) Sportartspezifische Leistungsdiagnostik im Kanu-Sport. Forschungsbericht, FKS. Leipzig.

75. Urhausen A, Coen B, Weiler B, Kindermann W (1994) Individuelle anaerobe Schwelle und Laktat steady state bei Ausdauerbelastungen. In: Clasing D, Weicker H, Böning D (eds). Stellenwert der Laktatbestimmung in der Leistungsdiagnostik. Stuttgart-Jena-New York: Fischer; Pp 37-46.

76. Urhausen A, Coen B, Weiler B, Kindermann W (1990) Sportmedizinische Leistungsdiagnostik und Trainingssteuerung in Rückschlagspielen. Leistungssport 20:29-34.

77. Urhausen A, Müller M, Förster HJ, Weiler B, Kindermann W (1986) Trainingssteuerung im Rudern. Dtsch Z Sportmed 37:340-346.

78. Vassiliadis A, Latour M, Mader A (1993) Entwicklung der Leistungsfähigkeit im Mittel- und Langstreckenlauf über ein Trainingsjahr. In: Martin D, Weigelt S (eds). Trainingswissenschaft. Selbstverständnis und Forschungsansätze; Sankt Augustin: Academia 1:217-225.

79. Vassiliadis A, Mader A, Hollmann W (1990) Zusammenhang von 4 (mmol/l) Schwelle, VO_2max und Wettkampfleistung bei Läufern von 800 m bis Marathon. In: Bernett P, Jeschke D (eds). Sport und Medizin – Pro und Contra; München; Zuckschwerdt; Pp 676-679.

80. Völcker K (1984) Probleme der Belastungsintensität beim Freizeitsport. Herz, Sport und Gesundheit 1:5-7.

81. Weber K, Gerisch G, Tritschoks HJ (1992) Leistungsphysiologische Aspekte zur Trainingssteuerung im Fußball. Kuhn W, Schmidt W (eds). Sankt Augustin: Academia; Pp 11-32.

82. Weineck J (1990) Optimales Training. Leistungsphysiologische Trainingslehre unter besonderer Berücksichtigung des Kinder- und Jugendtrainings. Erlangen: Perimed.

83. Zintl F (1988) Ausdauertraining. München-Wien-Zürich: BLV.

84. Zinner J, Pansold B, Buckwitz R (1993) Computergestützte Auswertung von Stufentests in der Leistungsdiagnostik. Leistungssport 23:21-26.

Performance diagnosis and training monitoring of human athletes in track & field running disciplines

Ulrich Hartmann and Margot Niessen
Institute for Movement and Training Science in Sports II, Faculty of Sport Science, University of Leipzig, Jahnallee 59, 04109 Leipzig, Germany; uhartmann@uni-leipzig.de

Introduction

Physiological running-specific performance ability is to a great extent determined by metabolic performance. During a running race of 1000 m (top time about 2:15 min) the average speed of male top elite athletes can be expected to be at about 7.58 m/s (27.27 km/h), during a 1500 m race (top time about 3:26 min) about 7.28 m/s (26.21 km/h), a heart rate (HR) of about 190-200 beats/min, a maximal relative oxygen uptake (VO_2max) around 76-78 ml/min/kg body weight (BW), a maximal post exercise blood lactate (LA) of about 16-12 mmol/l in the arterial blood after longer distances (1000 m, 1,500 m, 5,000 m) and of about 16-25 mmol/l after short and high intensive distances (100 m, 200 m, 400 m, 800 m) and a blood pH value between 7.0 and 6.85, representing the limit value of physiologically tolerable acidosis

A simple distribution of the energy requirement as proportions of the three existing energy resources (anaerobic alactic, anaerobic lactic and aerobic) can be calculated using the area pattern of proportional energy contributions (Hartmann, 1987).

Depending on the distance a high amount of the energy recruited during a competition is produced by the aerobic energy system, the rest is provided by the anaerobic lactic system and the anaerobic alactic nature (Hartmann, 1987; Hartmann and Mader, 1993). An overview on how energy can be quantified in different track and field events can be seen in Table 1.

Table 1. Share of energy supply in different track and field events of well trained athletes; further information see text.

Distance	ATP/CRPH (%)	Anaerobic-lac (%)	Aerobic (%)
30 m	80	19	1
60 m	55	43	2
100 m	25	70	5
200 m	15	60	25
400 m	12	43	45
800 m	10	30	60
1,500 m	8	20	72
3,000 m	5	15	80
5,000 m	4	10	86
10,000 m	3-2	12-8	85-90
Marathon	0	5-2	95-98

Metabolic background of energy supply in running disciplines

From the metabolic performance no direct inferences to competition velocity can be made, not even if a corresponding motivation during competition is taken into account. Elite athletes can use an excellent running technique to compensate for a lower metabolic performance only to some extent. Therefore, although a high metabolic performance is necessary, this is not a sufficient prerequisite for competition success.

Using the area calculation (Hartmann, 1987), statements about the development or the type of recruitment of the relevant proportions of energy provision are not possible. The reason for this is that, beyond the findings obtained, the really existent maximal aerobic performance (VO_2max) or the maximal lactic performance (glycolytic performance = maximal velocity of lactate development (VLAmax)) cannot be determined. Therefore it is absolutely necessary to measure oxygen uptake and post exercise blood lactate in laboratory (and if possible in field) and to calculate the metabolic background of the given load. Certain aspects of this problem will be discussed in more detail.

Figure 1 shows schematically the behaviour of VO_2 during the time course of a given load. From this graph also the importance of the VO_2 for the total energy supply of a running performance can be deduced. Generally it can be concluded that the area covered by the VO_2-uptake describes that portion of energy which is recruited aerobically. A general rule in load performance, and especially in running, is that a relative high portion of the necessary energy requirement is covered by the energy equivalent of the VO_2-uptake.

Because most of the energy of middle distance runners (800 m and longer distances) is produced by the aerobic energy system (see above) the determination of this portion is important to estimate the individual performance of a runner.

The formation of 1 mmol of ATP requires approx. 3.95 ml of O_2 (Di Prampero, 1981). The mitochondrial volume included in a normal red muscle fibre is about 3%, which corresponds to an O_2-uptake of the muscle of approx. 120 ml/min*kg (120*65/3.0 (see below) = 2,600 ml/min = 40 ml/min/kg of measured VO_2). In the case of a mitochondrial volume of approx. 6% in an endurance-trained runner (Hoppeler *et al.*, 1991; Mader *et al.*, 1988) this corresponds to an O_2-uptake of approx. 240 ml/min*kg (240*65/3.0 (see below) = 5,200 ml/min = 80 ml/min/kg of measured VO_2). The share of the working muscles in the body mass (active mass) is estimated at approx. 33%,

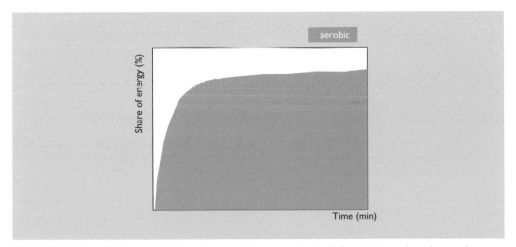

Figure 1. Schematic diagram of the influence of oxygen uptake (VO_2, dark area) to the total energy amount during a running competition. For further information see text.

while the total fluid volume (active and passive) is approx. 68-70% of the body mass, or about 47% as lactate distribution space (Mader, 1994; Mader and Heck, 1991). Taking into consideration these assumptions, there is a conversion factor between active muscle mass and body mass of approx. 3.0-3.1 for a runner weighing about 65 kg and having a VO_2max of approx. 5,400 to 5,600 ml/min or 77-80 ml/min*kg respectively (Hoppeler *et al.*, 1991; Mader *et al.*, 1988).

Admittedly, the energy supply recruited through the oxygen uptake alone (Figure 1) is not enough to meet the energy needs of the whole running competition (Figure 2). Especially in line with the starting power there is an enormous energy supply needed whereas the oxygen uptake is still increasing and accordingly an essential energy deficit exists. Therefore, shares of the energy supply have to be covered by anaerobic-lactic and anaerobic-alactic metabolic mechanisms pro-rata.

Besides the high oxygen uptake as gross criteria for the oxidative energy supply mechanism ($\geq$76 ml/kg), an accordingly high post exercise lactate value (16-18 mmol/l) is evidence for the importance of the anaerobic-lactic share for energy supply. The height of the lactate values is to some extent evidence for the glycolytic influence on the energy supply mechanism for particular running performances.

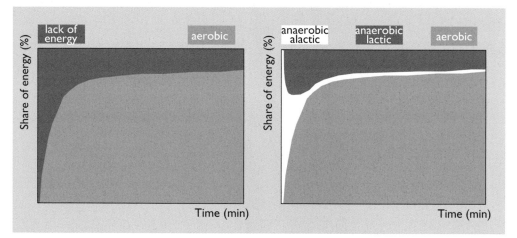

Figure 2. Schematic diagram of the total energy amount, divided in the VO_2 covered portion, and the other resources. For further information see text.

It must be pointed out that contrary to common opinion, the sole consideration or quantification of blood lactate provides unreliable information of the anaerobic-lactic or glycolytic share of energy supply. Table 2 clarifies the relationship of post exercise lactate concentrations in the blood and the calculated influence of the anaerobic energy supply. The estimation of the glycolytic share is considerably more difficult.

To estimate the so called 'maximal glycolytic' (anaerobic) performance it is necessary to estimate the (maximum) lactate formation rate (VLAmax)). The following example shows how the VLAmax for a not specific trained 100 m sprinter (time for 100 m running about 12 s, post exercise lactate about 14 mmol/l) and an experienced 400 m runner (time for 400 m about 44 s, post exercise lactate about 25 mmol/l) can be calculated:

12 s maximum load - 2 s free lactate load at the beginning = 12 - 2 s = 10 s maximal load; 14 mmol/l maximal post exercise blood lactate – 1.50 mmo/l blood lactate at rest = 12.5 mmol/l blood lactate netto
- (14 - 1.5) / (12 - 2) = 1.25 mmol/l*s VLA

Table 2. Share (%) of calculated anaerobic lactic energy supply, amount of post exercise blood lactate (mmol/l) and corresponding lactate formation rate (mmol/l*s) in different track and field events; further information see text.

Distance	Anaerobic-lac (%)	Blood-lactate (mmol/l)	VLAmax (mmol/l/s)
Rest	0.5	0.8-1.8	-
30 m	19	2-5	1.6
60 m	43	5-9	1.5
100 m	70	14-16-22	1.4-3.0
200 m	60	18-23	1.1-2.0
400 m	43	24	0.5-1.0
800 m	30	20	0.3-0.8
1,500 m	20	15	≈0.06
3,000 m	15	8-12	≈0.05
5,000 m	10	7-10	≈0.01
10,000 m	12-8	8	≈0.005
Marathon	5-2	3-4	≈0.0008

44 s maximum load - 2 s free lactate load at the beginning = 44 - 2 s = 42 s maximal load; 25 mmol/l maximal post exercise blood lactate – 1.50 mmol/l blood lactate at rest = 12.5 mmol/l blood lactate netto

- (25 - 1.5) / (44 - 2) = 0.56 mmol/l*s VLA

Figure 3 shows the behaviour of VLAmax for two different groups of athletes (short and long distance endurance runners) and given distances (30 to 400 m) on average. In general it is to be seen that the VLAmax is in the range of 0.6 and 1.0 mmol/l*s depending of the group and the distance (30 m/60 m); it is higher in that group which consists of more sprinters than more middle distance runners. This means that in correlation to the time the lactate production rate (VLA) is higher in the sprinters/short distance endurance athletes than in the long distance athletes. For very fast 100 m sprinters the VLAmax can be expected to be in the range of about 3.0 mmol/l*s, for middle distance runners in the range of about 0.5 mmol/l*s. The given findings make sense because of the increasing glycolytic influence on energy supply as shorter the competitive distance is and a decreasing VLA as longer the competition distance is.

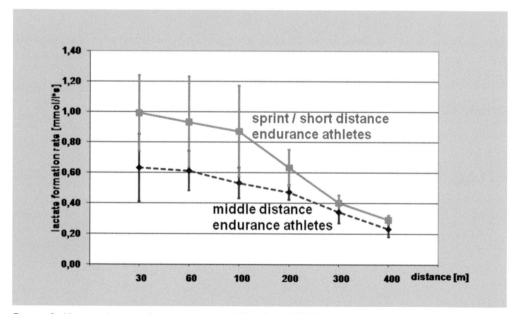

*Figure 3. Varying lactate formation rates (VLA (mmol/l*s)) for sprint/short distance endurance athletes and middle distance endurance athletes for different given distances; further information see text.*

If the increase of post-exercise blood lactate concentration (PBLC) by 14 mmol/l after a 1,500 m run is taken as the basis of the measurement, the net lactate formation is 0.06 mmol/l*s (14 mmol/l net PBLC)/(210 s exercise duration – 3 s lactate-free interval)). However, it would be wrong to assume that this very low rate of lactate formation calculated in the 1,500 m run corresponds to a sprinter´s VLAmax. The VLAmax of a fast 100 m runner, for example, is 1.0-1.4 mmol/l*s (Mader and Heck, 1991) or even higher (3.0 mmol/l*s) for a specific trained sprinter, depending of the individual glycolytic performance and adaptation level. However, inter-individual as well as intra-individual variabilities may be significant.

Because the glycolysis, or anaerobic-lactic share of energy supply, to provide maximum energy rates for covering the energy demand is not immediately available either, the first actions in a running competition must be recruited predominantly from available rich-in-energy phosphates.

Tests and testing procedures to determine individual human runner´s performance levels

For a differentiate examination and interpretation of endurance performance tests the following (practical) recommendations could be given:

1. Competition simulation test to acquire 'sport specific necessities'.
   This test is in accordance with the structure and duration of the sport specific competition load. It is to determine the sport specific performance and its individual limits.
   For middle distance runners (400 m, 800 m, 1000 m, 1,500 m) this is a 1 to 3 or 4 min maximum all out tests in accordance to the real competitive load. There is a focus in estimating the individual maximal speed, the discipline specific VO_2max, maximal blood lactate and also maximal heart rate. This test is to receive specific information about the metabolic background and the individual energy requirements.
2. Determination of the 'maximal oxidative' (aerobic) performance (VO_2max test).
   This test consists of multiple steps, each with a short duration and a rapid increase of the load (vita max test) to estimate the real and absolute VO_2max.

To determine maximal oxidative potential it is necessary to measure maximum oxygen uptake. In practice it is common to measure this by performing a stepwise increasing test (multiple increasing step test) but in reality this test does not provide the necessary valid data. Because of the duration of the whole test procedure (5 to 8 steps = 25 to 35 min) the fatigue of the tested athlete is increasing with the amount of steps; most often it is therefore not possible that an athlete performs at his real individual maximum exhaustion when he stops a further ongoing. That means by using this testing model an athlete will finish the test at his/her 'test specific exhaustion' level but not at their real individual limit of potential performance! According to the measurement of VO_2max this means that maximal VO_2 is underestimated by using a stepwise increasing test. In accordance to own results also VO_2 is measured about 200 to 400 ml lower that measuring it in a vita max test.

The vita max test on a treadmill should be performed as follows: warming up period in a very low speed (easy jogging) of about 10 min, after a 5 min resting time start at about 4.5 or 5.0 m/s; short duration (30 s) and rapid increase (0.5 m/s) of the steps without any break until total exhaustion. Measurement and determination of maximal speed, VO_2, lactate and heart rate.

3. Determination of the 'maximal glycolytic' (anaerobic) performance (estimation of lactate formation rate (VLAmax)).

   The test is characterised by a short duration, a supramaximal load for a very short time (5-10 s) for estimating the VLAmax.

   In practice and under traditional points of view the maximum post exercise lactate values are set equal to the so called maximum anaerobic capacity. But the fact is that the maximal lactate values do not provide any clear information about the anaerobic influence which is very much depends on multiple other factors as the level of performance/adaptation resp. the VO_2max, the load profile of the given discipline and others.

   The respective test is characterised by a short duration and a (supra)maximal load for a very short time (10-15 s). The higher the VLAmax the higher can the glycolytic influence be expected.

4. Determination of the endurance performance ability ('endurance capacity').

   This is the classical test procedure to determine endurance capacity of an individual. Ideally it consists of several steps of long duration (minimum 5 min, if possible even longer) and a small increase of the load; aim of this test is to estimate that what is called 'endurance' or those metabolic conditions which are close to the metabolic 'steady state/maxLass' (maximal lactate steady state) conditions.

The effect of an increase in endurance are schematically described in Figure 4). The saturation area of VO_2 of a 'normal' trained person increases from 65 to nearly 85% in a better trained individual (Figure 4, left graph). In the same time the accumulation of blood lactate as a marker for an increasing glycolytic influence is shifted to the right (Figure 4, right graph, dotted line). Compared to an untrained individual the beginning of the lactate accumulation increases to a 30 to 50% higher performance output value (Figure 4, right graph). This behaviour is the result of an increased oxidative influence (or a better oxidative performance) and a later and less intensive beginning glycolytic energy supply mechanism.

As a general test interpretation guideline we can summarise:

- A high anaerobic (glycolytic) performance is mostly combined with a low endurance performance (low 'aerobic capacity', bad threshold; 100 m sprinter).
- A high aerobic performance is mostly combined with a low glycolytic performance (or low lactate formation rate; marathon runner).
- The 'secret' for a high performance level in a given sport discipline (per example in running) is the 'correct' development of the different patterns of energy supply mechanisms at the 'right' time.

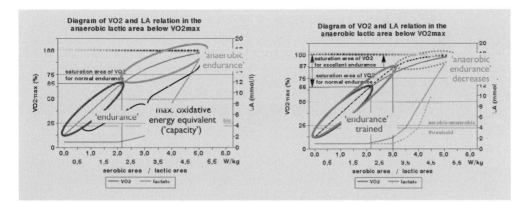

Figure 4. Relationship between oxygen uptake (VO_2 (%)) and blood lactate (mmol/l) during increasing load; for further information see text.

Training monitoring

Documentation of training data

In training science the relationship between load and recovery is the most important training principle. The former is quite dependent on the latter (e.g. Bompa and Jones, 1990; Hollmann and Hettinger, 2000); therefore, it is essential to collect and analyze exercise loads, both in time and content accurately (e.g. Reiß and Meinelt, 1985; Starischka, 1988; Keizer *et al.*, 1989; Röcker *et al.*, 1995; Martin and Coe, 2001). The analysis of load, recovery and performance depends on its precision of documentation. In literature most studies describe the simple average of intensity and weekly running training volume (e.g. Hagan *et al.*, 1981; Dotan *et al.*, 1983; Foster, 1983; Bale *et al.*, 1985; Svedenhag and Sjödin, 1985; Bale *et al.*, 1986; Brandon and Boileau, 1987; Sparling *et al.*, 1987; Marti *et al.*, 1988; Morgan *et al.*, 1989), but unfortunately only a few the specific distinction of training (various categories, zones and phases) (e.g. Liesen *et al.*, 1985; Föhrenbach, 1986; Badtke *et al.*, 1989, Vassiliadis *et al.*, 1993; Hewson and Hopkins, 1996; Martin *et al.*, 2001), specified in percentages of physiological parameters or indices (e.g. HR, LA; Föhrenbach, 1986; Vassiliadis *et al.*, 1993; Röcker *et al.*, 1995).

The following exercise data should be documented, recorded and analyzed:
- volume (VOL) like duration (h, min, s), distance (km, m), frequency (number of e.g. runs, lifts, jumps, throws etc.);
- intensities (INT) like HR (bpm), %HR_{max}, LA [mmol l^{-1}], velocity (v) (m s^{-1}, km h^{-1}) at 4 mmol l^{-1} LA (v_4);
- total amount of training, the running (RUN), the strength (STR) and the alternative (ALT) training; gross and net VOL; nowadays accelerometer based sensor technology among others (e.g. GPS devices, foot pods) make a real-time data-acquisition possible and support the objectivity of data (Niessen *et al.*, 2006).

The categorization of the detailed training data documentation is self-developed and based on specific code numbers of the German Track & Field Federation (Niessen, 2007):
- regenerative, compensatory training (REG) – ≤40 min (INT: ≤75% v_4);

- endurance I (extensive continuous) (E 1) – < 1.5 mmol l^{-1} LA (INT: ≤80% v$_4$);
- endurance II (intensive continuous) (E 2) – 1.5-3 mmol l^{-1} LA (INT: ≤90% v$_4$);
- endurance III (ext-/intensive intervals) (E 3) – 3-6 mmol l^{-1} LA (INT: ≥91% v$_4$);
- high Intensity Training (HIT) – >6 mmol l^{-1} LA (INT: ≥100% v$_4$);
- competition specific Training (CSZ) – high intensity and < 10 km;
- speed (Agility, Coordination) Training (S) – high intensity;
- strength Training (STR) – power lifting, resistance training, circuit training;
- alternative Training (ALT) – unspecific endurance training (e.g. cycling, etc.);
- competition (C) – variable intensity spectrum.

The statements to LA-zones refer to selective literature sources (e.g. Liesen *et al.*, 1985; Föhrenbach, 1986; Mader *et al.*, 1988; Mader and Heck, 1991; Foster *et al.*, 1993; Mader, 1994). The classification of RUN training methods is supported by a comparison with the individual, current performance diagnostic indices and largely in line with known applied physiologic classification schemes (Föhrenbach, 1986; Vassiliadis *et al.*, 1993; Niessen 1995). To comprehend and verify the exercise intensity, e.g in profiled terrain, in many cases LA and HR were determined. The loading rate during RUN training and competition was determined and used as a criterion for the mean current specific intensity (%INT v$_4$). Additional documented data both refer to passive and active resting times (e.g. breaks between exercises, sleep time) and recreation methods (e.g. sauna, physiotherapy).

Monitoring of load and recovery parameters

Nowadays a variety of different parameters along human biology and physiology support the monitoring process of track and field athletes.

Anthropometry and body composition

The loss of body weight is an indicator of catabolic processes in the human (Verma *et al.*, 1978) and animal muscle (Bruin *et al.*, 1994) and captured as an overload symptom in training documentation (e.g. Kuipers and Keizer, 1988; Lehmann *et al.*, 1993; Smith, 2000). As other causes there are also cellular fluid shifts (Kirwan *et al.*, 1988; O'Toole and Douglas, 1989), due to imbalance between water and electrolyte balance (Maughan *et al.*, 1989) or due to a high altitude stay (Hartmann *et al.*, 1994). The nutritional status and acute as well as chronic diseases are also mentioned as reasons for weight changes. As a very simple and routinely determined parameter the body weight can be individually collected almost daily. For detailed determination of the body composition (Ellis, 2000) nowadays often used methods are bioelectrical impedance and caliper measures.

Heart rate and heart rate variability under resting conditions

HR is subject to a complex regulatory network through modulation of the autonomic nervous system as well as local and systemic mediators (Israel *et al.*, 1974; Esperer, 1994) and is influenced by a variety of both exo- and endogene factors. Numerous field surveys described and discussed changes in HR and HR spectra (Abel *et al.*, 1993) under resting conditions (e.g. within the circadian rhythm during night) and in connection with endurance training (over)load-related symptoms (e.g. Israel, 1976; Bigger *et al.*, 1992; Esperer, 1992; Goldsmith *et al.*, 1997; Löllgen, 1999; Hedelin *et al.*, 2000; Berbalk and Bauer, 2001; Melanson and Freedson, 2001; Aubert *et al.*, 2003; Mourot *et al.*, 2004; Mourot *et al.*, 2004). One way to assess the situation of the ergotropic-trophotropic function in endurance athletes is to determine the long-term control of the cardiac chronotropic control at physical rest position, the heart rate variability (HRV). There is a risen HR due to an increased sympathetic tone and therefore decreased HRV. Time and/or frequency domain analysis monitored cardiac activities can be easily displayed and evaluated.

Hematological parameters: red and white blood counts

In elite sport there is a persistent interest in the determination of different, venous and/or capillary blood parameters, particularly red cell parameters (RBC), mainly due to the discussion on the effects of overload training and ergogenic aids (e.g. Ekblom and Berglund, 1991; Casoni *et al.*, 1993; Bodary *et al.*, 1999; Vergouwen *et al.*, 1999; Schmidt *et al.*, 2000). The variability of easy to determine RBC measures, like erythrocytes (Ery), hemoglobin (Hgb) and hematocrit (Hct), is associated with physiological (e.g. liquid balance; Schmidt *et al.*, 2000), environmental circumstances (Vergouwen *et al.*, 1999) and training itself (Bodary *et al.*, 1999; Schmidt *et al.*, 2000). Literature findings show data with relative broad spectra of variability and above respective limit values (Hgb, Hct) (e.g. Heath *et al.*, 1981; Hurtado *et al.*, 1945; Stegemann 1984; Sutton *et al.*, 1982). Therefore it is better to perform regular longitudinal RBC controls under strict standardized conditions to get an individual RBC-pattern ('fingerprint') and to prevent athletes with physiologically higher RBC levels from unpleasant consequences.

The immune system is one of the central functional systems, which affects the health and the performance significantly. It is in a steady area of conflict between training and competition intensity (e.g. stress stimuli in anaerobic metabolism, high psycho-physical performance pressure) and the summation of training stresses (e.g. Nieman, 2000). Physical work causes the proliferation of white blood cells, leukocytes (Leu). The behavior of the various elements of the leukocytes is distinguished in three phases (lymphocytic, neutrophilic and in-toxic phase) chronologically. Although it is difficult to measure the immunological status of athletes sufficiently objective, the longitudinal provisions of the Leu populations represents at least a trend.

Substrates and enzymes: creatine kinase, serum urea, muscle glycogen, anti-oxidative protection mechanism

Serum creatine kinase (CK) and serum urea (SU) are possible markers of muscular stress (CK) and catabolic protein degradation (SU) (e.g. Lemon and Nagle, 1981; Hortobagyi and Denahan, 1989; Hartmann and Mester, 2000). Both parameters support the detection of stress symptoms due to the extent and/or intensity of training regimes. Until now less detailed information about load-induced reactions in elite sports is known (e.g. Fabian *et al.*, 1989, 1992; Hortobagyi and Denahan, 1989). Individual rising of CK was detected immediately following loads with high intensity (e.g. middle distance event) or long duration exercise (e.g. marathon) (e.g. Hortobagyi and Denahan, 1989; Hartmann and Mester, 2000). On average CK- and SU-values of track and field athletes are within defined normal ranges, but with different inter- and intra-individual variability. Athletes with chronic low values only show a small variability, whereas athletes with chronic higher values had significant higher variance of the parameters. More running specific training tends to increase CK, more non-specific (e.g. cycling) to decrease SU. Due to a significant relation of blood SU and Hct a dependency to fluid balance can be assumed. In summary there exists inter-individual oscillations of CK (either frequency or amplitude) as well as inter- and intra-individual reactions of CK and SU due to overall training loads.

Training and competitive loads lead to a consumption of muscle glycogen in dependence of the intensity and duration of the exposure. Direct methods for its determination are ethically questionable (biopsy) or very expensive (NMR spectroscopy). The indirect determination through ammonia is a possible but also expensive blood parameter. Ammonia shows an opposite behavior to LA.

Numerous animal studies show a deleterious effect on muscle tissue of oxygen radicals during exercise. The number of investigations in humans is small and the findings are fragmentary. Glutathions are one of the most protective mechanisms against reactive oxygen (Heine *et al.*, 1995). A high priority is attached to glutathione-peroxidase, which is present in most body cells. It reduces hydrogen peroxide and other organic peroxides with simultaneous oxidation of glutathione (GSH). This means that the consumption of reduced glutathione (GSH) and the formation of oxidized glutathione (GSSG) is associated. GSH is regenerated by means of glutathione reductase and NADPH for GSSG. Numerous studies show that the concentration of GSH in the tissues is a reliable indicator of the balance between formation and decomposition of reactive oxygen derivatives. The glutathione-peroxidase has a low substrate specificity and degrades a variety of peroxides.

Metabolism-regulating hormones

It is assumed that the signal for recovery processes after physical stress is induced by the increasing amounts of metabolites, while a number of hormones enhance anabolic processes after stress (Jakovlev, 1977; Viru, 1985a; 1985b). Changes in hormone levels during the recovery phase have an importance for the speed of recovery processes and for the duration of the recovery phase (Kuipers and Keizer, 1988). The hormonal factors that are likely to be relevant in connection with the regulation of regeneration processes after physical stress, are the catecholamines (adrenaline and noradrenaline), the hormones of the hypothalamic-pituitary-adrenal axis (cortisol among others) and those of the hypothalamic-pituitary-gonadal axis (testosterone among others).

Psychological diagnostic tools: subjective stress profiles and diagnostics

The psycho-physical condition of athletes can be determined using a standardized recording sheet (e.g. Plath and Richter, 1978). It will examine whether there are visible differences in relation with the acute stress effect and compatibility before and after training. Stress effects are an expression of the interaction of the person, situation and action. They are also on the highest level of regulation of the intellectual processes and are reflected at the level of subjective experience. Individually different performance requirements lead to differences in the level of coping of the different stress states.

Resumee

In sport practice it is assumed that for each sport and discipline the performance limiting factors are well known, that an exact demand profile is established and also a plan of a performance build up is existent. But what exists are mostly phenomenological descriptions of the performance demand: for example the description of a 1000 m competitive race is mainly done with terms from training methodology and very rarely from physiology. Another example is the (wrong) opinion that high lactate values are an indicator for a high anaerobic 'capacity'. Those phenomenological based assumptions lead to unique views and self-fulfilling opinions in test interpretation and training methodology. Under the aspect of cyclization and periodization they have an important and unlucky influence on training schedules and programs.

Also many of the (common) laboratory test procedures and the way how they are used are partly or in total not fulfilling the basic quality criteria in performance testing! The 'simple' transfer of laboratory findings, as it exists in practice, is not very helpful and deserves an evaluation and sophisticated studies! But it would be necessary to give up the existing point of view and procedures, that with a single (metabolic) test many questions about the (correct) training load can be answered! This holds only as good as we are willing to evaluate continuously the existing points of view in a critical way!

References

Abel H-H, Koralewski HE, Krause R, Klüssendorf D, Droh R (1993) Ruhe-Monitoring der parasymphatischen Herzkontrolle: Vegetativer Status. In: Tittel K, Arndt KH, Hollmann W (eds). Sportmedizin: Gestern – heute – morgen. Bericht vom Jubiläumssymposium. Pp 133-137.

Aubert AE, Seps B, Beckers F (2003) Heart rate variability in athletes. Sports Med 33:889-919.

Badtke G, Giebel W, Israel S (1989) Sportmedizinische Grundlagen der Körpererziehung und des sportlichen Trainings. 2. Ed. Deutsch Harri. Leipzig, Germany.

Bale P, Rowell S, Colley E (1985) Anthropometric and training characteristics of female marathon runners as determinants of distance running performance. J Sports Sci 3:115-126.

Bale P, Bradbury D, Colley E (1986) Anthropometric and training variables related to 10 km running performance. Br J Sports Med 20:170-173.

Berbalk A, Bauer S (2001) Diagnostische Aussage der Herzfrequenzvariabilität in Sportmedizin und Trainingswissenschaft. In: Institut für Angewandte Trainingswissenschaft Leipzig (ed) 8.2. Aachen: Meyer & Meyer. Germany; Pp 156-176.

Bigger JT Jr, Fleiss JL, Steinman RC, Rolnitzky LM, Kleiger RE, Rottman JN (1992) Correlations among time and frequency domain measures of heart period variability two weeks after acute myocardial infarction. Am J Cardiol 69:891-898.

Bodary PF, Pate RR, Wu QF, McMillan GS (1999) Effects of acute exercise on plasma erythropoietin levels in trained runners. Med Sci Sports Exerc 31:543-546.

Bompa TO, Jones D (1990) Theory and methodology of training: the key to athletic performance. Dubuque, IO: Kendall & Hunt Pub. Co.

Brandon LJ, Boileau RA (1987) The contribution of selected variables to middle and long distance run performance. J Sports Med Phys Fitness 27:157-164.

Bruin G, Kuipers H, Keizer HA, Vander Vusse GJ (1994) Adaptation and overtraining in horses subjected to increasing training loads. J Appl Physiol 76:1908-1913.

Casoni I, Borsetto C, Cavicchi A, Martinelli S, Conconi F (1993) Reduced hemoglobin concentration and red cell hemoglobinization in Italian marathon and ultramarathon runners. Int J Sports Med 6:176-179.

Di Prampero PE (1981) Energetics of muscular exercise. Rev Physiol Biochem Pharmacol 89:144-222.

Dotan R, Rotstein A, Dlin R, Inbar O, Kofman H, Kaplansky Y (1983) Relationships of marathon running to physiological, anthropometric and training indices. Eur J Appl Physiol 51:281-293.

Ekblom B, Berglund B (1991) Effect of erythropoietin administration on maximal aerobic power. Scand J Med Sci Sports:88-93.

Ellis KJ (2000) Human body composition: *in vivo* methods. Physiol Rev 80:649-680

Esperer HD (1992) Herzfrequenzvariabilität, ein neuer Parameter für die nichtinvasive Risikostratifizierung nach Myokardinfarkt und arrhytmogener Synkopen. Herzschr Elektrophys 1:1-16.

Esperer HD (1994) Physiologische Grundlagen und pathophysiologische Aspekte der Herzfrequenzvariabilität beim Menschen. Herzschr Elektrophys 2:1-10.

Fabian K, Weber J, Schlegel D, Brenke H (1989) Das Isoenzym MB der Kreatinkinase (CK-MB) im Serum sportlicher Betätigung. Med Sport 29:142-145.

Fabian K, Schlegel D, Zerbes H (1992) Erfahrungen bei der Trainingssteuerung mit dem Parameter Serum Creatinkinase im Marathonlauf. Dtsch Z Sportmed 43:350-358.

Föhrenbach R (1986) Leistungsdiagnostik, Trainingsanalyse und -steuerung bei Läuferinnen und Läufern verschiedener Laufdisziplinen. Konstanz: Hartung-Gorre.

Foster C (1983) VO_2max and training indices as determinants of competitive running performance. J Sports Sci 1:13-22.

Foster C, Green MA, Snyder AC, Thompson NN (1993) Physiological responses during simulated competition. Med Sci Sports Exerc 25:877-882.

Goldsmith RL, Bigger JT, Bloomfield DM, Steinman RC (1997) Physical fitness as a determinant of vagal moderation. Med Sci Sports Exerc 29:812-817.

Hagan RD, Smith MG, Gettman LR (1981) Marathon performance in relation to maximal aerobic power and training indices. Med Sci Sports Exerc 13:185-189.

Hartmann U (1987) Querschnittsuntersuchungen an Leistungsruderern im Flachland und Längsschnittuntersuchungen an Eliteruderern in der Höhe mittels eines zweistufigen Tests auf einem GJESSING-Ruderergometer. Konstanz; Hartung-Gorre.

Hartmann U, Mader A1993) (Modelling of metabolic conditions in rowing through post-exercise simulation. Coach 4:1-15.

Hartmann U, Mader A, Glaser D, Burrichter H (1994) Veränderung von Parametern des roten Blutbildes bei Hochleistungsruderern im Rahmen eines Höhentrainings im Vergleich zum Flachland. In: Liesen H, Weiß M, Baum M (eds.). Regulations und Repairmechanismen. 33. Deutscher Sportärztekongress Paderborn 1993. Köln: Deutscher Sportärzte-Verlag.

Hartmann U, Mester J (2000) Training and overtraining markers in selected sport events. Med Sci Sports Exerc 32:209-215.

Heath D, Williams DR (1981) Man at high altitude. London, Melbourne, New York: Churchill Livingstone.

Hedelin R, Wiklund U, Bjerle P, Henriksson-Larsen K (2000) Cardiac autonomic imbalance in an overtrained athlete. Med Sci Sports Exerc 32:1531-1533.

Heine O, Dufeaux B, Kothe A, Prinz U, Rost R (1995) Bildung reaktiver Sauerstoffderivate und antioxidativer Schutz unter körperlicher Belastung: Übersicht Dt Z Sportmed 46:482-493.

Hewson DJ, Hopkins WG (1996) Specificity of training and its relation to the performance of distance runners. Int J Sports Med 17:199-204.

Hollmann W, Hettinger T (2000) Sportmedizin: Grundlagen für Arbeit, Training und Präventivmedizin. 4 Ed. Stuttgart, New York: Schatthauer Verlag.

Hoppeler H, Mathien-Costello O, Kayat SR (1991) Mitochondria and microvascular design. In: Crystal RG, West JB, Barnes PJ, Cherniak NS, Weibel ER (eds). The Lung; Raven Press; New York; Pp 1467-1477.

Hortobagyi T, Denahan T (1989) Variability in creatine kinase: Methodological, exercise, and clinically related factors. Int J Sports Med 10:69-80.

Hurtado A, Merino C, Delgado E (1945) Influence on the hemopaetic activity. Arch Intern Med 75:284.

Israel S, Kuppardt H, Gottschalk K, Neumann G, Böhme P (1974) Die submaximale Herzfrequenz als leistungsdiagnostische Kenngröße. Med Sport 14:297-304.

Israel S (1976) Zur Problematik des Übertrainings aus internistischer und leistungsphysiologischer Sicht. Med Sport 16:1-12.

Jakovlev NN (1977) Sportbiochemie. Leipzig: Barth.

Keizer H, Platen P, Menheere PPCA, Peters C, Wuest H (1989) The hypothalamic/ pituitary axis under exercise stress: the effects of aerobic and anaerobic training. In: Laron Z, Rogol AD. Hormones and Sport; Pp 101-115.

Kirwan JP, Costill DL, Mitchell JB, Houmard JA, Flynn MG, Fink WJ, *et al.* (1988) Carbohydrate balance in competitive runners during successive days of intense training. J Appl Physiol 65:2601-2606.

Kuipers H, Keizer HA (1988) Overtraining in elite athletes. Review and directions for the future. Sports Med 6:79-92.

Lehmann M, Foster C, Keul J (1993) Overtraining in endurance athletes: a brief review. Med Sci Sports Exerc 25:854-862.

Lemon PWR, Nagle FJ (1981) Effects of exercise on protein and amino acid metabolism. Med Sci Sports Exerc 13:141-149.

Liesen H, Ludemann E, Schmengler D, Föhrenbach R, Mader A (1985) Trainingssteuerung im Hochleistungssport. Dtsch Z Sportmed 36:8-18.

Löllgen H (1999) Herzfrequenzvariabilität. Dtsch Ärztebl 96:A 2029-2032.

Mader A (1984) Eine Theorie zur Berechnung der Dynamik und des steady state von Phosphorylierungszustand und Stoffwechselaktivität der Muskelzelle als Folge des Energiebedarfs. Köln: Deutsche Sporthochschule Köln.

Mader A (1994a) Aussagekraft der Laktatleistungskurve in Kombination mit anaeroben Tests zur Bestimmung der Stoffwechselkapazität. In: Clasing D, Weicker H, Böning D (Eds). Stellenwert der Laktatbestimmung in der Leistungsdiagnostik. Stuttgart, Jena, New York: Fischer; Pp 133-152.

Mader A (1994b) Die Komponenten der Stoffwechselleistung in den leichtathletischen Ausdauerdisziplinen – Bedeutung für die Wettkampfleistung und Möglichkeiten zu ihrer Bestimmung. In: Tschiene P (Hrsg.). Neue Tendenzen im Ausdauertraining. Informationen zum Leistungssport, Band 12 (Bundesausschuss Leistungssport). Frankfurt a. M.: Eigenverlag. PP 127-216.

Mader A, Hartmann U, Hollmann W (1988) Der Einfluss der Ausdauer auf die 6 minütige maximale anaerobe und aerobe Arbeitskapazität eines Eliteruderers. In: Steinacker JM (Ed.). Rudern: Sportmedizinische und sportwissenschaftliche Aspekte. Berlin, Heidelberg, London, Paris, New York, Tokyo: Springer; Pp 62-78.

Mader A, Heck H, Föhrenbach R, Hollmann W (1979) Das statische und dynamische Verhalten des Laktats und des Säure-BasenStatus im Bereich niedriger bis max. Azidosen bei 400-m und 800-m Läufern bei beiden Geschlechtern nach Belastungsabbruch. Dtsch Z Sportmed 30:203-249.

Mader A, Heck H (1991) Möglichkeiten und Aufgaben in der Forschung und Praxis der Humanleistungsphysiologie. Spectrum der Sportwissenschaft 3:5-54.

Marti D, Abelin T, Minder CE (1988) Relationship of training and life-style to 16-km running time of 4000 joggers. The '84 Berne 'Grand Prix' Study. Int J Sports Med 9:85-91.

Martin D, Carl K, Lehnertz K (2001) Handbuch Trainingslehre. 3. Ed. Schorndorf: Hofmann.

Martin DE, Coe PN (2001) Mittel- und Langstreckentraining. 3. Ed. Aachen: Meyer & Meyer.

Maughan RJ, Fenn CE, Leiper JB (1989) Effects of fluid, electrolyte and substrate ingestion on endurance capacity. Eur J Appl Physiol Occup Physiol 58:481-486.

Melanson EL, Freedson PS (2001) The effect of endurance training on resting heart rate variability in sedentary adult males. Eur J Appl Physiol 85:442-449.

Morgan DW, Baldini FD, Martin PE, Kohrt WM (1989)Ten kilometer performance and predicted velocity at VO_2max among well- trained male runners. Med Sci Sports Exerc 21:78-83.

Mourot L, Bouhaddi M, Perrey S, Cappelle S, Henriet MT, Wolf JP, *et al.* (2004a) Decrease in heart rate variability with overtraining: assessment by the Poincare plot analysis. Clin Physiol Funct Imaging 24:10-18.

Mourot L, Bouhaddi M, Perrey S, Rouillon JD, Regnard J (2004b) Quantitative Poincare plot analysis of heart rate variability: effect of endurance training. Eur J Appl Physiol 91:79-87.

Nieman DC (2000) Special feature for the Olympics: effects of exercise on the immune system: exercise effects on systemic immunity. Immunol Cell Biol 78:496-501.

Niessen M (1995) Verhalten von kardio-pulmonalen, metabolischen und spiroergometrischen Parametern während stufenförmig ansteigenden Belastungen auf dem Laufband bei Mittel- und Langstreckenläufern. Köln: Deutsche Sporthochschule Köln.

Niessen M, Hartmann H, Kinnunen H, Laukkanen R (2006) Accelerometer based sensor technology in running training. Med Sci Sports Exerc 38: S501.

Niessen M (2007). Determinanten von Belastung und Regeneration in Training und Wettkampf leichtathletischer Laufdisziplinen. Eine longitudinale, multifaktorielle Analyse anhand des Mittel- und Langstreckenlaufes. Tech. Univ. München. http://d-nb.info/988150883/34

O'Toole ML, Douglas PS (1989) The ultraendurance triathlete: physiologic and medical considerations. Med Sci Sports Exerc 21 (5 Suppl):S198-199.

Plath E, Richter P (1978) Der BMS(I)-Erfassungsbogen – Ein Verfahren zur skalierten Erfassung erlebter Beanspruchungsfolgen. Probleme und Ergebnisse der Psychologie 65:45-85.

Reiss M, Meinelt K (1985) Erfahrungen, Probleme und Konsequenzen bei der Erhöhung der Wirksamkeit der Steuerung und Regelung des Hochleistungstrainings. Theorie und Praxis Leistungssport 23:120-135.

Röcker K, Rieger J, Baumann I, Horstmann T, Dickhuth HH (1995) EDV-gestützte Trainingsanalyse in Synopsis zu leistungsdiagnostischen Daten am Beispiel Langstreckenlauf. In: Perl J, (ed.). Sport und Informatik IV. Berichte und Materialien des Bundesinstituts für Sportwissenschaft; Köln. Köln: Sport und Buch Strauß; Pp 53.

Schmidt W, Biermann B, Winchenbach P, Lison S, Boning D (2000) How valid is the determination of hematocrit values to detect blood manipulations? Int J Sports Med 21:133-138.

Smith LL (2000) Cytokine hypothesis of overtraining: a physiological adaptation to excessive stress? Med Sci Sports Exerc 32:317-331.

Sparling PB, Wilson GE, Pate RR (1987) Project overview and description of performance, training, and physical characteristics in elite women distance runners. Int J Sports Med 8 Suppl 2:73-76.

Starischka S (1988) Trainingsplanung. Schorndorf: Hofmann-Verlag.

Stegemann J. (1991) Leistungsphysiologie: physiologische Grundlagen der Arbeit und des Sports. 4th Ed. Stuttgart: Thieme.

Sutton JR, Jones NL, Houston CS (1982) Hypoxia: Man at altitude. New York: Thieme-Stratton.

Svedenhag J, Sjodin B (1985) Physiological characteristics of elite male runners in and off-season. Can J Appl Sports Sci 10:127-133.

Vassiliadis A, Latour M, Mader A (1993) Entwicklung der Leistungsfähigkeit im Mittel- und Langstreckenlauf über ein Trainingsjahr. In: Martin D, Weigelt S (eds.). Trainingswissenschaft. Selbstverständnis und Forschungsansätze. Sankt Augustin: Academia; Pp 217-225.

Vergouwen PC, Collee T, Marx JJ (1999) Haematocrit in elite athletes. Int J Sports Med 20:538-541.

Verma SK, Mahindroo SR, Kansal DK (1978) Effect of four weeks of hard physical training on certain physiological and morphological parameters of basket-ball players. J Sports Med Phys Fitness 18:379-384.

Viru A (1985a) Hormones in muscular activity, Vol. I: Hormonal ensemble in exercise. CRC Press Inc., Boca Raton.

Viru A (1985b) Hormones in muscular activity, Vol. II: Adaptive effect of hormones in exercise. CRC Press Inc., Boca Raton.

Practical news on advances in nutrition for performance horses and ponies between 2009-2011

Véronique Julliand[1] and Sarah L. Ralston[2]
[1]URANIE-USC 'Nutrition of the Athletic Horse', AgroSup Dijon, 26 bvd Dr. Petitjean, BP 87999, 21079 Dijon cedex, France; v.julliand@agrosupdijon.fr
[2]Rutgers, the State University of New Jersey, Dept. Animal Science, 84 Lipman Drive, New Brunswick, NJ 08901, USA

Introduction

Nutrition of equine athletes is critical to their performance, health, well-being and longevity. Despite differences in the concerns among the various disciplines (i.e. racing versus jumpers versus endurance), many areas are of general concern, such as glucose/insulin metabolism, energy and protein intake, types of feeds, feed management in relation to performance, supplements and stimulants of various types. The objective of this paper is to critically review the most recent scientific literature with respect to potential changes in recommendations for nutritional management of performance horses.

Glucose/insulin metabolism

Factors influencing glucose/insulin metabolism and responses have been the topic of over 33 studies in just the past year. It is becoming increasingly obvious that there are so many factors that influence glucose/insulin concentrations responses in horses that data even from well-controlled studies are hard to evaluate. Indeed, the safety and validity of the most recently accepted tests of insulin sensitivity and resistance are in question and need further investigation.

The 'gold standard' blood evaluation tests questioned

The 'gold standard' to evaluate insulin sensitivity and glucose metabolism in recent years has been the insulin modified frequently sampled intravenous glucose tolerance test (iFSIGT) or other high dose intravenous challenges such as the hyperinsulinemic euglycemic clamp test and associated 'proxies' calculated from a single fasting glucose/insulin sample. They have been used extensively in experimental studies (see below) and even diagnostically (Durham *et al.*, 2009) to detect insulin resistance and/or abnormalities or changes in glucose disposition. However, in the past two years the sensitivity and validity of these non-physiologic challenges and interpretation of a single blood sample analyzed for just glucose/insulin ('proxies') have been questioned:

- It appears that the glucose/insulin doses used in the iFSIGT challenges should be reduced to 100 mg glucose/kg BW (instead of 300; Toth *et al.*, 2009) to avoid the confounding effect of glucosuria (loss of glucose in the urine) on the results.
- The same research group reported that plasma insulin alone is not a good measure of 'pancreatic beta cell function' as commonly used in the 'proxies'. They concluded that connecting peptide (C-peptide), which is secreted by the pancreas concurrently with insulin but that does not undergo hepatic degradation and clearance, should be measured at the same time (Toth *et al.*, 2010). This is because insulin hepatic clearance may be reduced in some cases of insulin resistance, independent of the higher pancreatic secretory activity in response to challenges, contributing to higher, more prolonged plasma insulin concentrations that do not reflect true pancreatic beta cell activity.
- Most studies utilizing the recommended 20 mIU insulin infusion in the iFSGIT have utilized unfit and/or insulin resistant horses without reports of adverse effects. The use of that dose, however, in iFSGITs administered to lean (average body condition score of 2/5), fit Standardbred horses resulted in clinically apparent hypoglycaemia that necessitated administration of intravenous glucose (Barton *et al.*, 2011).
- The use of intravenous infusion 'clamp' studies that cause extreme elevations (>1000 mIU/l) of plasma insulin by 5 to 48 hr has well been documented to alter uptake of glucose and fatty acids by skeletal muscle and alter glucose transporters (Suagee *et al.*, 2011) and to reliably induce laminitic changes (deLaat *et al.*, 2010) even in clinically normal horses. However, the relevance of these conditions to the physiologic elevations recorded in naturally occurring insulin resistance (usually <500 mIU/l for no more than 1 or 2 hours after a high starch meal or dextrose challenge) is unclear.

The use of a single dose of insulin (20 to 50 mu/kg/BW) in fasted, normal horses with only four blood samples being drawn during the challenge (as opposed to over twenty in the iFSIGT) proved to be a repeatable, sensitive and reportably safe measure of insulin sensitivity in both normal and insulin-resistant, unfit light-breed horses (Caltibilota *et al.*, 2010; Earl *et al.*, 2011) and could potentially be applied under field conditions However, the safety and efficacy of this challenge has yet to be determined in fit horses.

The limitation of single blood sample evaluations

Testing horses for insulin resistance, whether or not they are experiencing any clinical signs of metabolic disorders, has become popular in recent years. However it is very important to recognize that if only a single, so called 'fasting' sample is taken for interpretation that there are a myriad of factors that can cause elevations in glucose, insulin or both that may be misinterpreted. For example, previous drug treatments should be taken into consideration. Haffner *et al.* (2009) reported that a single dose of 40 mg/kg BW dexamethasone initially (2 & 24 hr) resulted in reduced insulin sensitivity but at 72 hr there was a rebound effect, possibly due to cortisol suppression. Injection of epinephrine, simulating a stress condition, also blocked the effect of an insulin injection on plasma glucose concentrations (Earl *et al.*, 2011), essentially creating insulin resistance.

Mature Arabian horses consistently had higher insulin responses to a wide variety of processed feeds fed at the rate of 1.5 g/kg BW than did two-year olds under the same management (Nielsen *et al.*, 2011). In a study comparing low protein (650 g protein/d) to high protein (1,600 g protein/day) intakes in adult, fit Standardbred horses using the iFSGIT and 'proxies' showed no dietary effect on the standard measures of the minimal model analysis but the low protein horses exhibited more rapid and prolonged clinical hypoglycaemia following the insulin injection that could have been due to leaner body mass or metabolic fitness (Barton *et al.*, 2011). Therefore, in addition to taking into consideration the feed to which the horse was adapted (see below), time and content of the last meal when evaluating a single sample of blood glucose/insulin, it is also important to consider the effect of stress, age and degree of physical fitness.

Despite repeated previous reports of seasonal and diurnal variation in apparent insulin sensitivity in horses in both the northern and southern hemispheres, Place *et al.* (2010) reported no seasonal variation in serum insulin or glucose concentrations but instead a higher resting concentration of adrenocorticotropic hormone (ACTH) in a field study of 9 'normal' and 10 laminitic horses residing on a single farm in Missouri, USA in August-October relative to other months. However 5/9 of the 'normal' horses had body condition scores of 7/9 or higher despite no history of laminitis or evidence of 'endocrinopathies' and the laminitic horses were undergoing dramatic dietary modifications over the course of the study. In addition the blood samples used were not truly fasting samples, being drawn between 08:00 and 11:00 h from horses that had access to grass hay. The evidence for both seasonal and diurnal variation in insulin sensitivity remains strong and therefore should also be considered if evaluating a single or even multiple blood samples.

The role of leptin is unclear

The insulin resistance commonly associated with obesity in horses may also be associated with high plasma concentrations of leptin, a hormone that is associated with control of appetite (Caltibilota *et al.*, 2010). Carter *et al.* (2009) found that increasing BCS from an average of 6/9 to 8/9 in adult Arab or Arab cross horses (by feeding a 60% sweet feed/40% forage/roughage ration that provided 156-193% of NRC requirements for horses at maintenance) did not alter resting glucose but caused significant hyperinsulinemia (compensated insulin resistance) and hyperleptinemia. Hyperinsulinemia has been repeatedly documented previously to be associated with both obesity and prolonged feeding of high starch/sugar rations but the association with high plasma leptin is relatively new. The researchers were utilizing the iFSGIT and 'proxies' to assess glucose/insulin responses and noted that there was a large amount of individual variation in the insulin responses, especially as the horses got to peak obesity. However, Van Weyenberg *et al.* (2010) reported instead an improvement in apparent glucose tolerance associated with elevated plasma leptin in horses supplemented with carnitine, so the correlation between leptin and glucose tolerance/insulin resistance is still not clear.

Reduction of obesity, diet restriction and related endocrinopathies

In a follow up study on the obese horses created by Toth *et al.* (2009), use of low to moderate exercise for 5 weeks without dietary restriction did reduce body weight but there was no change in the insulin sensitivity parameters being assessed (Carter *et al.*, 2010). Both control and exercised horses were on alfalfa/grass mix hay at 2.5% BW with 1 kg of grain based concentrate daily. There was an increase in resting insulin in both treatments that could have been a seasonal response and also there was a high degree of individual variability that would have caused lower statistical power and obscured potential benefits. An exercise regimen that was equivalent to the low intensity training in the study above (3 days/wk for 15 weeks at 60% maximum heart rate for 30 min), was reported to significantly improve insulin sensitivity in normal, previously sedentary young and old Standardbred mares but the ration was not described (Liburt *et al.*, 2011).

Overweight ponies fed 1% body mass in the form of a nutritionally balanced, chaff based ration lost 1% of their initial body mass per week, predominantly as fat reduction, over 12 weeks (Dugdale *et al.*, 2010). The ration was divided into two daily feedings and no adverse health effects (i.e. Hyperlipidemia or hepatic dysfunction) were observed. However the ponies ate more rapidly and were more active in their stalls during the period of restriction relative to when they had had free access to the feed before the study, during which time they consumed on average 2.5% body mass per day. Only 3/5 of the ponies were hyperinsulinemic at the onset of the restriction, and by the end of the 12 weeks only one was mildly hyperinsulinemic (44 mu insulin/l plasma). Body condition scores did not correlate well with the measured reductions in body mass and body fat. The conclusion was that feeding a balanced, forage based ration providing 8.5 MJ/kg DM at the rate of 1% body mass (on a dry matter intake basis) was a safe and effective way to reduce body weight in ponies.

The role of the diet

The now common assumption that large high starch/sugar meals for horses are to be avoided is also being drawn into question. Tinworth *et al.* (2011) confirmed that horses adapted to high starch rations tended to have higher and more rapid insulin secretion in response to challenges, commonly interpreted as insulin resistance (Borgia *et al.*, 2010) but also documented improved disposal, so the apparent hyperinsulinemia in grain-adapted horses was actually fairly transient and adaptive and not near the excessively high and prolonged plasma insulin concentrations used to reliably induce laminitis experimentally (>1000 mu/ml for over 36 hours; de Laat *et al.*, 2010). Gordon *et al.* (2011) also reported that feeding 3.6 kg textured grain mix (29.4% fat, 10.6% sugar, 5% fat, 6.5% fiber) /day with 1% BW moderate quality grass hay had no prolonged adverse effects on insulin sensitivity in young horses relative to those fed the same amount of a high fat/ fiber grain-based concentrate (16.6% starch, 3.7% sugar, 9.5% fat, 13% fiber). Vervuert *et al.*, (2009a) however, pointed out that insulin responses to a meal of grain were much more variable than glycemic responses.

Thermal processing of corn significantly increased its glycemic impact relative to cracking or pelleting but it was also noted that reduced glycemic response, such as seen with cracked corn, may reflect incomplete digestion/absorption of the starches present that would potentially result in starch bypass of the small intestine and cause large intestinal fermentative disruptions (Nielsen *et al.*, 2010). Therefore simply reducing the glycemic response to a meal may not, in the long run, be desirable.

Feeding strategies will also affect glucose/insulin measurements. Despite some recommendations that horses can be offered hay before taking 'resting' blood samples, forages can significantly impact plasma insulin. Horses given 8 hours of access to fescue pastures had significant increases in plasma insulin and glucose reflecting the diurnal fluctuation in starch content of the grasses (Sharlette *et al.*, 2011). The pastures used in that study varied from 13.5% NSC at 08:00h to 19% NSC at 20:00h. The horses turned out from 07:00h-15:00h had lower plasma insulin on average than when turned out from 12:30h-20:00h when the NSC was highest. This study reinforced the recommendation that metabolically challenged horses be allowed pasture access only in the morning hour when grass NSC is lowest. If horses are fed a single meal of concentrate/day in the morning they will have higher glucose insulin responses if fed hay 15 min before the concentrate meal than if the hay was fed after the grain was presented or if the total amounts feed were spread out over 2 or 3 feedings (Saul *et al.*, 2011). The use of obstacles such as bocce balls or grated inserts placed in feed buckets will slow feed intake and reduce postprandial insulin peaks (Kutzner-Mulligan *et al.*, 2011).

There are many supplements being marketed to purportedly improve insulin sensitivity and reduce hyperinsulinemic responses in horses. There were no benefits detected to the addition of fish oil (324 mg oil/kg BW/day) to the ration of mares in light exercise (Hoffman *et al.*, 2011). The lower area under the curve for the glycemic responses to the supplemented and control meals of grain observed was probably due to the fact that the amount of grain fed with oil was reduced to keep the rations isocaloric. Similarly Earl *et al.* (2011) failed to detect any benefit of supplementing hyperleptinemic, hyperinsulinemic mares with fish oil (10 ml twice a day) top dressed on textured sweet feed or dosing the mares with cinnamon extract. Vervuert *et al.* (2010) also failed to detect any benefit to the supplementation of either fish oil (0.2 ml/kg BW) or soybean oil (0.2 ml/kg BW) added to cracked corn fed at the rate of 2 g Starch/kg BW to normal horses. Supplemental leucine (0.05 to 0.2 g/kg BW) had no effect on glycemic responses to a meal of grain (Etz *et al.*, 2011), though all doses significantly increased plasma leucine but decreased plasma isoleucine and valine, a potentially detrimental effect. Chameroy *et al.* (2011) also failed to detect any benefit of supplementation of chromium (5 mg/day) and magnesium (8.8 mg/day) in a yeast based supplement top dressed on 0.25 kg oats fed to previously laminitic obese horses, 12/14 of which had compensated insulin resistance.

Psyllium (90 g/day) fed with a hay (1.5% BW mixed grass) and commercial whole grain concentrate (0.5% BW) ration for 60 days did reduce both postprandial glucose and insulin responses to a meal of the concentrate and to an IV dextrose challenge (10% dextrose infused at 0.5% BW after an overnight fast; Moreaux *et al.*, 2011). Increasing the dose of psyllium to either 180 or 270 g, however, did not significantly increase the effects on glucose metabolism so it is unclear if an even lower dose may have been effective.

Tinworth *et al.* (2010) found that chronic daily administration of metformin (15 mg/kg per os twice a day) had poor bioavailability that would limit its usefulness as a therapeutic drug in ponies. Durham *et al.* (2010) used metformin in combination with glibenclamide, pergolide and dietary alterations to successfully restore normoglycemia in 3 cases diagnosed by iFSIGT to have type 2 Diabetes mellitus, but it is not clear which of the drugs used in combination with diet changes were responsible for the improvements observed.

Energy recommendations

There are many resources available that give energy and nutritive values for different feedstuffs as well as horse energy requirements and recommendations for feeding. In Europe the different feeding systems used are based on digestible energy (DE), metabolizable energy (ME), or net energy (NE). Each of these systems has some limitations that are currently the subject of research and the German system has recently been reviewed (Coenen, 2011).

New tools for measuring energy requirements for exercised horses

There are limitations in the accuracy of most energy requirement recommendations. In the French energy system (INRA, 1990) four work categories (very light, light, moderate and heavy) were defined for exercised horses. From data provided with saddle and leisure horses these categories were based on the utilisation type (indoor or outdoor), on the daily duration of the activity and on its intensity estimated with the different gaits used during the exercise. However the activity provided (intensity, length and frequency) at a similar work level varies highly depending on the discipline (flat racing, harness racing, jumping, endurance, etc.). In the United States the National Research Council (NRC) 2007 recommendations for the four categories of effort (light, moderate, heavy and very heavy) were also based on the average duration of the daily work and its intensity but intensity was evaluated by the average heart rate (HR) measured during the exercise (NRC, 2007). For example, for the category 'very high', the average weekly duration of exercise can vary from one to twelve hours with very high or low speeds at average HR between 150 and 110 beats/minute respectively during the exercise. However the recommendations still need refinement to better evaluate intensity, especially in anaerobic work.

Recent works have explored new methodologies to measure the intensity of energy expenditure (EE) of exercising horses. New perspectives have been opened thanks to the validation of a new portable device consisting of a respiratory mask (Equimask) and a portable respiratory gas analyser (K4b2) which allows field measurements of volume of oxygen consumption (VO_2) in exercising horses (Art *et al.*, 2006). The aerobic exercise intensity can be estimated by measuring VO_2 that reflects the requirement for ATP by muscle activity via oxidative processes. Cottin *et al.* (2010) measured VO_2 and carbon dioxide production (VCO_2) using the K4b2 on Arabian horses during a track exercise test at increasing speeds up to 12.5 m/s. Similarly a continuous incremental exercise test was conducted on a racetrack with French trotters harnessed to a sulky equipped with the K4b2 system (Goachet *et al.*, 2011). The velocity reached at the last completed step went up to 11.1 m/s. In both studies, the portable devices were successfully used: the mask was well accepted by the horses and the data obtained were comparable to reference values obtained with a fixed respiratory gas analyser on a treadmill.

Another way of measuring exercise intensity is to record heart rate (HR) which has been proven to be highly correlated to VO_2 (Coenen, 2008). HR can be recorded by commercially available instruments under practical conditions during any type of exercise. Coenen (2010) considered HR to be a very accurate reflection of exercise intensity because this is a biological signal that integrates both intrinsic (breed, body weight, individual muscle fiber profile, etc.) and extrinsic (rider's capability, track surface, temperature, etc.) factors. In Australia, heart rate was monitored to quantify the energy expenditure (EE) of horses during the four periods of a polocrosse game (Buzas *et al.*, 2009). Those measurements were used to calculate that the horses had an average EE of 0.55 ± 0.124 MJ Net Energy (NE) per minute of play. Also the authors could discriminate among horses playing in position 1 (attack) which tended to have higher rates of energy expenditure than those playing in position 2 (center) or 3 (defence). In Italy a similar study was conducted with horses competing in 3 day eventing (dressage, jumping and cross-country) either at the expert or intermediary level (Valle *et al.*, 2009). For the intermediate levels, the EE was estimated to average 3.76, 2.24 and 4.44 MJ NE for dressage, jumping and cross-country competitive efforts, respectively. For the expert levels, the average EEs were 3.01, 2.42 and 6.19 MJ NE for the same events, respectively.

Using VO_2 or HR data allows a first estimation of EE for different types of exercise. However the EE estimation further needs to take into account whether the activity is aerobic or anaerobic and add in the oxygen debt for an anaerobic effort. Indeed as soon as the ATP synthesis is anaerobic, VO_2 does not accurately reflect the energetic expenditure (Coenen *et al.*, 2011) and nor does the use of HR.

This is why Coenen (2010) has suggested the use of blood lactate concentration to establish anaerobic EE. When exercise intensity increases, blood lactate levels increase also, indicating a higher contribution of anaerobic energy metabolism to total EE. Based on the caloric equivalent for accumulated lactate, a lactate accumulation of 1 mmol/min is equivalent to 1.03-1.8 J/sec of expended energy. As an example, for a horse with 5.8 mmol lactate at HR 180, an anaerobic contribution to total energy expenditure of 18 and 46% could be expected for HR of 200 and 220, respectively (Coenen, 2010).

Another method recently studied was the use of maximal aerobic speed (MAS), which is the velocity corresponding to the achievement of VO_2max, to quantify the horse effort. Goachet *et al.* (2011) evaluated a new test protocol to determine the MAS during a driven trotting exercise.

The model of miniature horses into question

Miniature horses (MH) are sometimes used as models for exercised horses. Therefore it is of interest to know how comparable they are relative to larger horses. Legere *et al.* (2011) evaluated them in standardised exercised tests and compared their physiological responses to those of Quarter Horses (QH) performing the same tests. They detected no differences in heart rate responses to the tests which were equivalent to submaximal training between MH and QH. However hematocrit, haemoglobin and red blood cells were lower in MH than in QH during increasing speeds, peak, completion and recovery period suggesting differences between breeds as models and putting the use of MH as models into question.

New equations for estimating nutritive values of feeds

A major way to determine horse feedstuff nutritive value is to evaluate its energy content. Whereas NRC (2007) relies on the digestible energy (DE), the German group is currently developing new feeding standards based on metabolizable energy (ME) because this is the way nutritional energy is expressed in most other domestic species (Coenen *et al.*, 2011). In addition to faecal energy losses, ME takes into account gas losses due to fermentation (primarily methane) and urine losses, which in horses are higher than methane. By using regression analysis, Kienzle and Zeyner (2010a, b) predict that:

- Mean methane energy loss is of 0.002 MJ/g crude fiber (CF) intake. The authors mentioned that hindgut fermentation in horses relies probably more on acidogenesis than does ruminant fermentation.
- Mean urinary energy loss from the digestion and absorption of energy from hay is 0.008 MJ/g crude protein (CP) intake. The authors concluded that using CP was more accurate than using digestible crude protein (DP), which overestimated the renal losses for hay compared to concentrates. The presumed reason was that many aromatic compounds, in particular the phenolic acids of forage cell-walls, can be metabolized in the gut and conjugated into hippurate (a carboxylate) which is absorbed and excreted in urine, falsely elevating the organic energy source losses.

Therefore the new equation to predict ME that is proposed in the German system is:

ME (MJ/kgDM) = -3.54 + 0.00129 CP + 0.0420 crude fat - 0.0019 CF + 0.0185 N-free extract.

With: N-free extract = Dry Matter% - (CP% + crude fat% + CF%)
Crude nutrients in g/kg DM

This equation, however, is not applicable for feeds or forages with >10% crude fat.

Starch and fibre intake recommendations

The management of equine nutrition cannot ignore the use of thresholds for intake of nutrients that guarantee that the ration is complete and will not adversely affect the animal. The main focus currently is on fibre and starch intake.

Regarding the roughage intake, Coenen *et al.* (2011) recommend at least 20 g roughage (84% to 90% DM) per kg BW per day, which is twice the previous one. This recommendation for forage was based on behaviour and digestive health considerations but it is not exact. The authors recommend to take into account the quality of forage: if high quality forages are used the recommended intake can indeed exceed the amount of energy required by horses with low energy requirements and result in undesirable weight gain.

As for starch intake, Geor (2010) reminded that individual meals should not contain more than 2.0 g starch/kg BW for optimization of starch digestion within the small intestine and minimization of gastrointestinal disturbances associated with the flow of undigested starch to the large intestine. Nonetheless, the new recommendation is that a starch intake should not exceed 1.1 g/kg BW/meal (Coenen *et al.*, 2011). Feeding starch over that threshold has been associated with a higher risk for the development of gastric ulceration syndrome (EGUS) in Denmark (Luthersson *et al.*, 2009). However this epidemiological study did not confirm a direct cause-effect between starch feeding and EGUS and it is possible that other dietary factors such as a low structural fibre intake contributed to this apparent association (Luthersson *et al.*, 2009). Coenen *et al.* (2011) recommend a meal size of 0.3 kg/100 kg BW for compound feeds or grains with a starch content of between 30 and 40%. Even further limitation is necessary in feedstuffs with starch levels exceeding 40%. The relation between starch intake and insulin metabolism is variable and has been discussed in a previous part of the present review.

Data should be interpreted very cautiously because to date starch intake and structural fibre intake have often been confounded by simultaneous alterations: generally an increase in meal starch content is associated with a decrease in fibre content, and it is difficult to determine which factor had contributed to observed changes.

Feed digestibility

Impact of processing of feeds

Processing of feeds, whether cereals or hays, can dramatically affect their digestibility and nutritive values. Mature geldings fed popped milo, whole oats or rice bran in a 60:40 ratio with coastal Bermuda grass hay had dramatically higher starch but lower fat apparent digestion on the popped milo relative to the others (Winchell *et al.*, 2011) but it was also noted that the rice bran treatment significantly reduced calcium retention (Winchell TL, in verbal presentation 2011). Thermal processing of corn increased digestibility relative to feeding whole or mechanically processed corn or oats, however it was pointed out that the more rapid and higher increases in postprandial glucose absorption may be desirable, indicating more complete digestion of starches/sugars in the small intestine to avoid bypass of the highly fermentable carbohydrates to the large intestine (Nielsen *et al.*, 2010).

Due to differences in the chemical structure, hydrophilic balance, and particle size of insoluble fibres, the type and processing methods of roughages can alter both water hydration capacity and potential water releasing capacity in horses, which can potentially impact hydration during strenuous activity (Parsons *et al.*, 2011). Water hydration capacity was positively correlated with neutral detergent fiber content in a comparison of alfalfa hay, grass hay, beet pulp and a fiber mix of chopped hays and soyhulls. Five mm particle size samples had a higher WHC and EPWRC than 1 mm samples. The potential for water release, however, was greatest in grass hay and lowest for the fiber mix, with alfalfa hay and beet pulp being equally intermediate (Parsons AM, verbal communication in presentation, 2011) suggesting that long grass hays might be more beneficial in competitions where hydration status over time is of significant concern than beet pulp or alfalfa based roughages or mixes.

New factors brought into consideration for digestibility of exercised horses

Ponies were used as models for horses at maintenance in many trials for measuring the apparent digestibility of feedstuffs. Despite the important role in many competitive activities, they have not been used in exercise associated digestibility studies mainly run with horses. Longland *et al.* (2011) showed the DM and GE digestibilities of complementary feeds were significantly greater than those of the hay in exercised ponies and that the DM digestibilities were considerably higher than that reported for exercised Thoroughbreds fed similar diets. Further work should determine whether there are significant differences in the digestibility of complementary feeds by physically fit, exercised ponies and horses.

Breeds can differ in their ability to digest their rations and thus to maintain weight and condition on a given feed. Ragnarsson and Jansson (2010) documented that Standardbreds were unable to maintain body weight when fed haylages that caused weight gain in Icelandic horse fed at the same rate and under the same conditions, despite having comparable apparent digestion of nutrients. Jensen *et al.* (2010) however, found that Icelandic horses had significantly higher apparent digestibility of most nutrients (crude fiber, dietary fiber and starch) in a haylage/concentrate ration than did Danish Warmbloods fed the same rations.

Knowledge of the impact of both exercise and physical activity on digestion is essential to adapt the feeding practices to horses in training and competition. Goachet *et al.* (2010) assessed the influence of long-term endurance conditioning on cell wall digestion in horses. They showed that digestibility coefficients of neutral detergent fibre were significantly higher after 10 weeks of training, corresponding to the 90 km level, and tended to be higher after 17 weeks conditioning to reach 120 km level. The authors suggested that this increase could be beneficial for endurance horses as it would provide more energy from forage degradation.

Protein

A new concept for protein supply and requirement

With regard to what is known in other species, there is a great concern in equine nutrition for developing new concepts for more precise protein requirements: the theoretical ideal protein is defined by the balance of the essential amino-acids for the horse, which are not well defined. Feeding the ideal amount of protein, with no deficiency or excess, necessitates understanding the metabolic availability of the limiting amino acids and relative digestibility of the protein source.

The German group defines both the neutral detergent insoluble crude protein (NDICP) and the neutral detergent soluble crude protein (NDSCP) according to the Cornell Net Carbohydrate and Protein System for cattle (Coenen *et al.*, 2011). This allows discrimination between cell wall protein, which cannot be broken down by autoenzymatic digestion, and cell content protein which may be digested by enzymes in the small intestine (Coenen *et al.*, 2011).

It is considered in equines that the majority of the amino-acids are absorbed from the small intestine and that the amino-acids originated from the microbial fermentation in the hindgut play a negligible role. It was found recently that the equine proximal colon expressed specific amino-acid transporters of the brush-border membrane in similar abundance than that of the jejunum suggesting that it might contribute to both cationic and neutral amino-acids uptake and absorption (Woodward *et al*, 2010). Another *in vitro* study provided strong evidence for significant L-lysine uptake by the large colon showing that, on a per gram tissue basis, L-lysine uptake capacity in the large colonic mucosal layer was 78% that of the distal jejunal mucosal layer (Woodward *et al.*, 2011). Further studies are necessary to determine whether the hindgut derived microbial proteins contribute to whole body homeostasis via large intestinal absorption, as it is the case in the pigs.

Exercise impacts protein and amino-acids requirements

The impact of conditioning and exercise on the protein and amino acid requirements also has become an issue.

Additional muscle mass is gained via muscle hypertrophy during conditioning which may impact the nitrogen (N) balance in exercising horses. In a study where crude protein intake was kept as constant as possible (1.9 g/kg BW) and exercise intensity was held constant, N balance improved with conditioning, due to the reduction of urinary nitrogen loss (Graham-Thiers and Bowen, 2011a). Since there was no difference in fecal nitrogen loss, these data suggested that horses were making more efficient use of the protein that was digested and absorbed. However the authors could not conclude whether the additional retained N was due to a specific metabolic need or to support additional muscle mass.

Intense exercise over a distance of 2000 m influenced the concentrations of most plasma amino-acids in trotters compared to the basal level taken before the effort (Hackl, 2009). Whereas some plasma concentrations (alanine, aspartate, glutamate, isoleucine, leucine, lysine and taurine) increased, others (arginine, asparagine, citrulline, glutamine, glycine, histidine, methionine, serine, tryptophan and 3-methylhistidine) decreased after exercise or remained constant (ornithine, threonine, tyrosine, phenylalanine and valine). The intensity of the exercise also impacted some plasma amino-acids concentrations: at higher exercise intensities tryptophan concentration decreased and taurine increased. The authors suggested that these changes could reflect shifts between the free amino-acid compartments, but there were also some indications for muscle catabolism.

Specifying protein diets for exercised horses

Nitrogen balance of exercising horses fed different diets were evaluated by Graham-Thiers and Bowen (2011b). Horses were fed five different CP intakes on a BW basis (1.4, 1.5, 1.6, 1.7 and 1.8 g/kg BW). Nitrogen retention (NR) was higher and the urine urea-N index was lower for horses fed 1.6 g CP/kg BW compared to the four other diets. This was also the case when NR was expressed on a BW basis. The authors concluded that the diet which appeared to be the best for N retention as well as the most efficient use of protein (1.6 g CP/kg BW) was close to the recommendation given by the current NRC (NRC, 2007). In another study (Graham-Thiers and Bowen, 2011c), horses received similar amounts of crude protein from either grass hay (840 g) or hay plus grain (865 g). Despite the similar amounts of crude protein intake, some plasma amino-acid concentrations (methionine, valine, lysine, phenylalanine, arginine) were increased in horses fed hay plus grain compared with the hay only group, reflecting likely the increased foregut digestibility as well as a greater quality amino-acid profile in the grain. There was also improved nitrogen balance in the hay plus grain group, presumably due to the higher availability of amino-acids.

The impact of a high fibre and a high starch diet was compared in moderately trained Dutch warmblood horses (Alberghina *et al.*, 2010). Plasma serotonin and pH were significantly higher in horses fed a high fibre diet than those fed a high starch diet. The higher serotonin reflects higher tryptophan availability from forages and purportedly may have a calming effect. Higher blood pH may reduce the adverse acidogenic effects of intense exercise.

Essen-Gustavsson *et al.* (2010) compared the influence of two high energy forage-only diets providing a high crude protein intake (16.6%) versus recommended (12.5%) on muscular glycogen and free pool amino-acid concentrations taken before and after intense exercise in Standardbred horses. They showed that muscle glycogen and leucine concentrations in the muscle of horses post training were higher with the high crude protein intake. Urschel *et al.* (2011) also documented that feeding a 33% protein supplement (2 g/kg BW) at 0 and 30 min after an 18 hour fast promoted indices of muscle protein synthesis. It may be beneficial for muscle recovery to feed horses more crude protein than the current recommendations during intense training.

Supplements

It is becoming increasingly popular to supplement horses with amino-acids and/or minerals on the empirical supposition that they might be deficient in the ration. The use of single amino-acids has been generally assumed to be 'safe' however this might not necessarily be true.

Malesky *et al.* (2011a) documented that supplementation of 2 times the recommended requirement of lysine to sedentary adult geldings fed a corn-based concentrate (60% of total), lysine deficient ration resulted in significant decreases in total plasma non-essential amino-acids and especially in the essential amino-acids, methionine and threonine. The authors suggested that the decreases in methionine and threonine were perhaps due to increased skeletal muscle uptake but it could also have been a reduction in absorption, though there was no overall reduction in total nitrogen retention.

Concern with vitamin/mineral deficits leading to reduced immune function or oxidant damage is also common. Adult, sedentary horses fed 70% of daily recommended Se intake (LS group; <0.06 ppm selenium in total ration) for 28 days had lower whole blood selenium and glutathione peroxidase relative to both pre-trial values and to horses (AS) fed 140% the recommended daily selenium intake and a higher ratio of triiodothyronine to thyronine in the LS horses suggested borderline or incipient selenium deficit (Brummer *et al.*, 2011a). However blood selenium and glutathione peroxidase also decreased in the AS horses and the indices of oxidative stress measured (serum total anti-oxidant capacity and serum malondialdehyde) did not differ between the two groups. The LS horses did have a delayed and reduced immune response to a novel vaccine (Bummer *et al.*, 2011b) but no other indices of immune function were altered relative to AS horses. White *et al.* (2011) also found no benefit to supplementation of selenium as sodium selenite in excess of recommendations (0.3 mg Se/Kg DM versus control: 0.1 mg Se/kg DM) to sedentary horses but reported a slight decrease in oxidative damage in unconditioned mares subjected to 120 min of submaximal exercise (25.8 km at walk/trot, mean heart rate 135 beats/min) relative to controls. Haggert *et al.* (2010) reported that higher blood Se concentrations were not associated with improved performance in horses competing in endurance competitions in California. Plasma selenium concentrations did not differ between horses that completed a ride and those that were disqualified for metabolic failure or lameness, although blood Se concentrations were higher in horses that were reported to have received oral Se supplementation.

References

Alberghina D, Giannetto C, Visser EK, Ellis AD (2010) Effect of diet on plasma tryptophan and serotonin in trained mares and geldings. Vet Rec 166:133-136.

Art T, Duvivier DH, van Erck E, de Moffarts B, Votion D, Bedoret D, Lejeune JP, Lekeux P, Serteyn D (2006) Validation of a portable equine metabolic measurement system. Eq Vet J Suppl 36: 557-561.

Barton KD, Foote CE, Cawdell-Smith AJ, Anderson ST, Boston RC, Bryden WL (2011) Dietary Protein level and glucose and insulin dynamics in mature geldings. Recent Adv Anim Nutr Australia 18:97-98.

Borgia LA, Valberg SJ, McCue ME, Pagan JD, Roe CR (2010) Effect of dietary fats with odd or even numbers of carbon atoms on metabolic response and muscle damage with exercise in Quarter Horse-type horses with type 1 polysaccharide storage myopathy. Am J Vet Res 71:326-336.

Brummer M, Hayes S, Earing JE, McCown SM, Lawrence LM (2011a) Effect of selenium depletion on oxidative stress in mature horses. J Eq Vet Sci 31:257.

Brummer M, Hayes S, Earing JE, McCown SM, Adams AA, Horohov DW, Lawrence LM (2011b) Selenium depletion reduces vaccination response in horses. J Eq Vet Sci 31:266.

Buzas AM, Cawdell-Smith AJ, Dryden G McL, Bryden WL (2009) Physiological responses and energy expenditure of polocrosse horses during competition. J Eq Vet Sci 29:303-304.

Caltibilota TJ, Earl LR, Thompson DL, Clavier SE, Mitcham PB (2010) Hyperleptinemias in mares and geldings: Assessment of insulin sensitivity from glucose responses to insulin injection. J Anim Sci 88:2940-2949.

Carter RA, McCutcheon LJ, George LA, Smith TL, Frank N, Geor RJ (2009) Effects of diet-induced weight gain on insulin sensitivity and plasma hormone and lipid concentrations in horses. Am J Vet Res 70:1250-1258.

Carter RA, McCutcheon LJ, Valle E, Meilahn EN, Geor RJ (2010) Effects of exercise training on adiposity, insulin sensitivity, and plasma hormone and lipid concentrations in overweight or obese, insulin-resistant horses. Am J Vet Res 71:314-321.

Chameroy KA, Frank N, Elliott SB, Boston RC (2011) Effects of a supplement containing chromium and magnesium on morphometric measurements, resting glucose, insulin concentrations and insulin sensitivity in laminitic obese horses. Eq Vet J 43:494-499.

Coenen M (2008) The suitability of heart rate in the prediction of oxygen consumption, energy expenditure and energy requirement of the exercising horse. In: M Saastomoinen, W Martin-Rosset (eds). Nutrition of the exercising horse. Wageningen: Wageningen Academic Publishers; Pp 139-146.

Coenen M (2010) Remarks on the Benefits of Heart Rate Recordings. Feeding and veterinary management of the sport horses. Proc Kentucky Eq Res; Pp 42-54.

Coenen M, Kienzle E, Vervuert I, Zeyner A (2011) Recent German developments in the formulation of energy and nutrient requirements of horses and the resulting feeding recommendations. J Eq Vet Sci 31:219-229.

Cottin F, Métayer N, Goachet AG, Julliand J, Slawinski J, Billat V, Barrey E (2010) Oxygen consumption, gait variables and running economy of Arabian endurance horses measured during a field exercise test. Eq vet J 42 Suppl 38:1-5.

De Laat MA, McGowan CM, Sillence MN, Pollitt (2010) Hyperinsulinemic laminitis. Vet Clin North Am Eq Pract 26:257-264.

Dugdale AH, Curtis GC, Cripps P, Harris PA, Argo CM (2010) Effect of dietary restriction on body condition, composition and welfare of overweight and obese pony mares. Eq Vet J 42:600-610.

Dugdale AH, Curtis GC, Cripps P, Harris PA, Argo CM (2010) Effect of dietary restriction on body condition, composition and welfare of overweight and obese pony mares [Erratum appears in Eq Vet J 2011 43:121] Eq Vet J 42:600-610.

Durham AE, Hughes KJ, Cottle HJ, Rendle DI, Boston RC (2009) Type 2 diabetes mellitus with pancreatic beta cell dysfunction in 3 horses. Eq Vet J 4:924-929.

Earl LR, Thompson DL, Mitcham PB (2011) Factors affecting the glucose response to insulin injection in mares: Epinephrine and supplementation with cinnamon extract or fish oil. J Eq Vet Sci 31:249-250.

Essen-Gustavsson B, Connysson M, Jansson A (2010) Effects of crude protein intake from forage-only diets on muscle amino acids and glycogen levels in horses in training. Eq Vet J 42 Suppl 38:341-346.

Etz LC, Lambert NM, Sylvester JT, Urschel KL, Staniar WB (2011) Supplemental leucine's influence on plasma glucose, insulin and amino acid responses in Quarter Horse yearlings. J Eq Vet Sci 31:248-249.

Geor RJ (2010) Digestive strategy and flexibility in horses with reference to dietary carbohydrates. In: AD Ellis, AC Longland, M Coenen, N Miraglia (eds). The impact of nutrition on the health and welfare of horses. Wageningen: Wageningen Academic Publishers; Pp 37-39.

Goachet AG, Varloud M, Philippeau C, Julliand V (2010) Long-term effects of endurance training on total tract apparent digestibility, total mean retention time and faecal microbial ecosystem in competing Arabian horses. Eq Vet J 42 Suppl 38:387-392.

Goachet AG, Fortier J, Julliand V, Assadi H, Lepers R (2011) The use of equine K4b2 during incremental field exercise tests in driven Standardbred trotters: a preliminary study. In this book.

Gordon MB, Jerina ML, Raub RH, Williamson KK(2011) Insulin sensitivity in growing horses fed higher starch versus higher fat diet for two years. J Eq Vet Sci 31:277-278.

Graham-Thiers PM, Bowen LK (2011a) The effect of conditioning on nitrogen balance in exercising horses. J Eq Vet Sci 31:272-273.

Graham-Thiers PM, Bowen LK (2011b) Using urinary urea-N as an assessment of protein requirements and protein quality in exercising horses. J Eq Vet Sci 31:273-274.

Graham-Thiers PM, Bowen LK (2011c) Effect of protein source on nitrogen balance and plasma amino acids in exercising horses. J Anim Sci. 89:729-735.

Hackl S, van den Hoven R, Zickl M, Spona J, Zentek J (2009) The effects of short intensive exercise on plasma free amino acids in standardbred trotters. J Anim Physiol Anim Nutr 93:165-173.

Haffner JC, Eiler H, Hoffman RM, Fecteau KA, Otiver JW (2009) Effect of a single dose of dexamethasone on glucose homeostasis in healthy horses by using the combined intravenous glucose and insulin test. J Anim Sci 87:131-135.

Haggett E, Magdesian KG, Maas J, Puschner B, Higgins J, Fiack C (2010) Whole blood selenium concentrations in endurance horses. Vet J 186:192-196.

Hoffman RM, Kayser JP, Lampley RM, Haffner JC. (2011) Dietary fish oil supplementation affects plasma fatty acids and glycemic response but not insulin sensitivity. J Eq Vet Sci 31:252-253.

Husted L, Sanchez LC, Baptiste KE, Olsen SN (2009) Effect of a feed/fast protocol on pH in the proximal equine stomach. Eq Vet J 41:658-662.

INRA (1990) L'alimentation des chevaux. W Martin-Rosset (ed), INRA, Paris ; Pp 232.

Jensen RB, Brokner C, Knudsen KE, Tauson AH (2010) A comparative study of the apparent total tract digestibility of carbohydrates in Icelandic and Danish warmblood horses fed two different haylages and a concentrate consisting of sugar beet pulp and black oats. Arch Anim Nutr 64:343-356.

Kienzle E, Zeyner A (2010a) Metabolizable energy for horses: development of a simple and flexible feed evaluation system. In: AD Ellis, AC Longland, M Coenen, N Miraglia (eds). The impact of nutrition on the health and welfare of horses. Wageningen: Wageningen Academic Publishers; Pp 37-39.

Kienzle E, Zeyner A (2010b) The development of a metabolizable energy system for horses. J Anim Physiol Anim Nutr 94:doi: 10.1111/j.1439-0396.2010.01015.x

Kienzle E, Zeyner A, Coenen M (2010) Der Erhaltungsbedarf von Pferden an umsetzbarer energie. Übersichten Tierernährung 38:33-54.

Kutzner-Mulligan J, Hewitt K, Sharlette J, Smith J, Pratt-Phillips S (2011) The effect of different feed delivery methods on rate of feed consumption and serum insulin concentration in horses. J Eq Vet Sci 31:300

Legere RM, Arns MJ, Pendergraft JS (2011) Heart rate and hematology response to submaximal training in quarter and miniature horses. J Eq Vet Sci 31:233-234.

Liburt NR, Fugaro MN, Wunderlich EK, Zambito JL, Horohov DW, Betancourt A, Boston RC, McKeever KH, Geor RJ (2011) Effect of exercise training on insulin sensitivity and muscle tissue cytokine profiles of old and young Standardbred mares. J Eq Vet Sci 31:237-238.

Longland AC, Barfoot C, Harris PA (2011) The apparent digestibility of hay and concentrate feeds by exercised ponies. J Eq Vet Sci 31:274-275.

Luthersson N, Nielsen KH, Harris P, Parkin TDH (2009) Risk factors associated with equine gastric ulceration syndrome (EGUS) in 201 horses in Denmark. Eq Vet J 182:67-72.

Malesky SM, Chen L, Löest CA, Turner JL (2011) Plasma amino acid response in mature geldings fed three concentrations of Lysine. J Eq Vet Sci 31:255-256.

Moreaux SJJ, Nichols JL, Bowman JGP, Hatfield PG (2011) Psyllium lowers blood glucose and insulin concentrations in horses. J Eq Vet Sci 31:160-165.

NRC (2007) Nutrient Requirements of horses. Washington DC. Sixth edition. National Academic Press. Washington, DC.

Nielsen BD, O'Connor-Robison CI, Spooner HS, Shelton J (2010) Glycemic and insulinemic responses affected by age of horse and method of feed processing. J Eq Vet Sci 30: 249-258.

Parsons AM, Nielsen BD, Schott HC, Geor R, Yokoyama M, Harris P (2011) Effects of fiber type, particle size, and soak time on water hydration and estimated potential water releasing capacities of roughages fed to horses. J Eq Vet Sci 31:261.

Place NJ, McGowan CM, Lamb SV, Schanbacher BJ, McGowan T, Walsh DM (2010) Seasonal variation in serum concentrations of selected metabolic hormones in horses. J Vet Internal Med 24:650-654.

Ragnarsson S, Jansson A (2010) Comparison of grass haylage digestibility and metabolic plasma profile in Icelandic and Standardbred horses. J Anim Physiol Anim Nutr DOI: 10.1111/j.1439-0396.2010.01049.x

Saul JL, Nyhart AB, Reddish JM, Alman M, Cole K (2011) Effect of feeding practice on glucose, insulin, and cortisol responses in Quarter Horse mares. J Eq Vet Sci 31:299.

Sharlette J, Hewitt K, McLeod SJ, Fellner P, Siciliano P (2011) Effect of pasture consumption on blood insulin, glucose and volatile fatty acid concentration in horses. J Eq Vet Sci 31:298-299.

Suagee JK, Corl BA, Hulver MW, McCutcheon LJ, Geor RJ (2011) Effects of hyperinsulinemia on glucose and lipid transporter expression in insulin-sensitive horses. Domestic Anim Endocrin 40:173-181.

Tinworth KD, Edwards S, Noble GK, Harris PA, Sillence MN, Hackett LP (2010) Pharmacokinetics of metformin after enteral administration in insulin-resistant ponies. Am J Vet Res 71:1201-206.

Tinworth KD, Raidal SL, Harris PA, Sillence MN, Noble GK (2011) Comparing Glycaemic and insulinaemic reponses of ponies and horses to dietary glucose. J Eq Vet Sci 31:301.

Toth F, Frank N, Elliott SB, Perdue K, Geor RJ, Boston C (2009) Optimization of frequently sampled intravenous glucose tolerance test to reduce urinary glucose. Eq Vet J 41:844-851.

Toth F, Frank N, Martin-Jimenez T, Elliot SB, Geor RJ, Boston RC (2010) Measurement of C-peptide concentrations and responses to somatostatin, glucose infusion and insulin resistance in horses. Eq Vet J 42:149-155.

Urschel KL, Escobar J, McCutcheon LJ, Geor RJ (2011) Effect of feeding a high-protein diet following an 18-hour period of feed withholding on mammalian target of rapamycin-dependent signaling in skeletal muscle of mature horses. Am J Vet Res 72:248-255.

Valle E, Odore R, Badino P, Girardi C, Zanatta R, Bergero D (2009) Use of GPS and heart rate monitoring system to assess the effort during the eventing competitions. Proc New findings in equ pract. Centro Internazionale del Cavallo. Druende (TO); Pp 49-53.

Van Weyenberg S, Buyse J, Janssens GP (2009) Increased plasma leptin through l-carnitine supplementation is associated with an enhanced glucose tolerance in healthy ponies. J Anim Physiol Anim Nutr 93:203-208.

Vervuert I, Voigt K, Hollands T, Cuddeford D, Coenen M (2009) The effect of mixing and changing the order of feeding oats and chopped alfalfa to horses on: glycaemic and insulinaemic responses, and breath hydrogen and methane production. J Anim Physiol Anim Nutr 93:631-638.

Vervuert I, Voigt K, Hollands T, Cuddeford D, Coenen M (2009) Effect of feeding increasing quantities of starch on glycaemic and insulinaemic responses in healthy horses. Vet J 182:67-72.

Vervuert I, Klein S, Coenen M (2010) Short-term effects of a moderate fish oil or soybean oil supplementation on postprandial glucose and insulin responses in healthy horses. Vet J 184:162-6.

White S, Warren LK, Bobel J (2011) Effects of dietary selenium and exercise on antioxidant enzyme activity in equine blood and skeletal muscle. J Eq Vet Sci 31:266-267.

Winchell TL, Baker LA, Pipkin JL, Brown MS, Lawrence TE, Robbins R (2011) *In vitro* starch digestibility of various grains and digestibility of popped milo, rice bran and whole oats in mature geldings. J Eq Vet Sci 31:260.

Woodward AD, Holcombe SJ, Steibel JP, Staniar WB, Colvin C, Trottier NL (2010) Cationic and neutral amino acid transporter transcript abundances are differentially expressed in the equine intestinal tract. J Anim Sci 88:1028-33.

Woodward AD, Fan MZ, Steibel JP, Geor RJ, Taylor NP, Trottier NI (2011) Characterization of D-glucose transport across equine jejuna brush border membrane using pigs as an efficient model of jejunal glucose uptake. J Eq Vet Sci 31:280-281.

Zeyner A, Kirchhof S, Susenbeth A, Südekum KH, Kienzle E (2010) Protein evaluation of horse feed: a novel concept. In: AD Ellis, AC Longland, M Coenen, N Miraglia (eds). The impact of nutrition on the health and welfare of horses. Wageningen: Wageningen Academic Publishers; Pp 37-39.

Do animals use natural properties of plants to self-medicate?

Sabrina Krief
Departement Hommes, Natures, Sociétés UMR 7206, Muséum National d'Histoire Naturelle, 57 rue Buffon, 75005 Paris, France; krief@mnhn.fr

For more than 30 years, field studies have shown that chimpanzees ingest items of low nutritional value such as rough leaves, bitter stems of *Vernonia amygdalina* and clay, apparently thereby protecting themselves against parasites and renforcing their health. Among animals, several species of insects and birds as well as other mammals have been evidenced to use secondary compounds to recover or to maintain health. Recently, we described the diversity and the biological activities of items of low nutritional value used by wild chimpanzees in Uganda suggesting a broad repertoire of natural substances that our closest relatives are able to use.

Use of secondary metabolites of plants by different animal species

Insects

Some invertebrates have overcome the chemical barrier of noxious plants products. Insects can for example use plants secondary compounds in their antipredator strategy or as selfmedication by sequestering saponins or alkaloids, caterpillars later use them to kill endoparasites (Termonia *et al.*, 2002). A recent study shows that the fitness of parasited wooly bear caterpillars (*Grammia incorupta*) was improved when they had the opportunity to use a synthetic food containing pyrrolizidine alkaloids. When uninfected, the fitness is reduced by the consumption of this diet. The caterpillars adapted their foraging choice differently according to their parasited status (Singer *et al.*, 2009). The mechanism to explain such ingestion has been explored: a specific taste alteration appears when caterpillars get infected by parasites, increasing the likelihood that the caterpillars will feed on usually unpalatable plants that can provide chemical defenses (Bernays and Singer, 2005). However, the female behavior of oviposition is determinant for the survival of descendants: in a lab experiment, Lefevre *et al.* (2010) found that female monarchs infected with parasites showed a strong preference for laying their eggs on top of a special variety of milkweed plant (*Asclepias currasavica*) in which the total content in cardenolides is 17-fold higher than in the other *Asclepia* species available. Uninfected female monarchs, however, showed no preference between the two species. The adult butterflies cannot cure themselves with the plant, but they can alleviate the disease in their offsprings in choosing to lay eggs on it. This is likely the first report to demonstrate medication process that targets a conspecific rather than the sick consumer itself.

Parasitism is even a higher burden in social animals especially insects that live in the same nests for several generations thus having a low genetic diversity. This can facilitate the spread and the adaptation of parasites to the hosts. Wood ants (*Formica paralugubris*) collect pieces of solidified resin from coniferous trees known to inhibit the growth of bacteria and fungi in ants nest material (Christe *et al.*, 2003). The use of such material is lead by odour cues and is prophylactic rather than curative (Chapuisat *et al.*, 2007).

Birds

Birds such as *Sturnus vulgaris* are also well known to incorporate in their nest aromatic plants that can inhibit the growth of bacteria and inhibit ectoparasite growth (Clark and Masson, 1985 and 1988). Olfaction was shown to be a major feature for the selection of herbal medicine in Blue tits in Corsica (Petit *et al.*, 2002). Another way suggested to play a major role in the control of ectoparasites – or symptoms they produced – in birds is the application of ants in the feather known as «anting» behavior (Clayton, 1999).

Mammals

External uses of plants has been also described in mammals: fur-rubbing is practiced with resin (white-nose coatis; Gompper and Hoylan, 1993), aromatic plants (capuchins monkeys; Baker, 1996) or millipeds after having bitten them (Birkinshaw, 1999). Several explanations are proposed to explain such behaviors: besides the major one being to reppel insects or parasites, a role as social facilitator is not excluded.

A study conducted on 215 faeces of leopards collected in Ivory Coast revealed that more than 10% out of them contained grass (Hoppe-Dominik, 1988). In addition, these carnivores – as chimpanzees – swallowed the hispid grass without chewing it. Authors did not investigate a possible relationship with parasitism.

Dogs are also well known to eat grass and the reason frequently proposed to explain this behaviour is their mechanic emetic effect. However, three different studies failed to find out a relationship between a pathologic status and the grass eating in dogs studied (Sueda *et al.*, 2008; Bjone *et al.*, 2007 and 2009; Mc Kenzie *et al.*, 2010).

Individual learning was experimentally evidenced in domesticated sheep (Villalba *et al.*, 2006). During conditioning, diseases are induced through special diets provided together with the medication. After this phase, sick sheep are able to select the correct antidote and to recover while sheep that were not conditioned were unable to select the medication. This capacity of associating disease with a medication was also tested in other domestic species. A PhD study conducted in USA tested four chronically lame horses to examine their ability to associate a flavour (carrots or apples), with a possible post-ingestive physiological consequence induced by a drug (Williams, 2008). Two drugs were tested: swainsonine from locoweed and butorphanol tartrate, a synthetic opiate analgesic (Torbugesic™). The toxin swainsonine is known to cause the neurological disorder described as locoism in large continuous doses sometimes leading to the death of horses. Some reports suggested it might act as an addictive substance (as the synthetic opioate analgesic) explaining the consumption by horses despite its noxious effect. Each group of two horses was assigned a respective drug throughout the duration of two separate trials. The first trial associated a flavour with each group's respective drug treatment and the second trial involved the reversal of flavours while holding the drug treatments constant for each group. Each trial involved a conditioning period followed by test days when horses were challenged to make a decision between the treatment-associated flavour or the non-treatment-associated flavour. In the first trial all horses preferred the non-treatment diet whatever the associated flavour. In the second trial the horses that can choose the opiate preferred the drug diet while the other ones still fed on the non-treatment diet. The results of this study suggest that horses do have the ability to associate a taste with a post-ingestive effect induced by a drug and supports the hypothesis that horses may have selected the opiate to reduce the pain. Nevertheless, the associative process for wild animals facing a wide diversity of natural products in dynamic interaction with predators, pathogens, and climatic stress is a very high challenge compared to select diets proposed for experimental studies.

In great apes

Records on uses of rough leaves for deworming were first observed decades ago (Wrangham and Nishida, 1983). They suggested that this is likely a common behaviour in African apes: 34 plant species were recorded to be used for their mechanical effect by chimpanzees, bonobos and lowland gorillas (Huffman and Wrangham, 1994). Consumption of bitter pith of *Vernonia amygdalina* was a first evidence of chemical activities of plants ingested (Huffman and Seifu, 1989). However, phytochemical studies have only been carried out on a single species, *Vernonia amygdalina* and apart from the mechanical effect of rough leaves, recorded evidences of self-medicating behaviour in chimpanzees were still rare until we started to combine phytochemistry with data on chimpanzee ecology and health.

Plants eaten by chimpanzees contain bioactive compounds

In Kibale National Park, Uganda, I monitor the chimpanzee (*Pan troglodytes schweinfurthii*) diet since 1999. The collaborative work between Ugandan institutions – Makerere University (MU) and Uganda Wildlife Authority (UWA) – and French ones – MNHN and ICSN-CNRS – has enabled to achieve the collection of a large part of plant species eaten by the Kanyawara chimpanzees (parts consumed and not consumed). A total number of 400 extracts of the 480 Ugandan plant parts collected have already been screened against different targets (systemic parasites, tumoral cells, etc) to evaluate their bioactivities. Out of them, some are rarely consumed and have a low nutritive value. We thus explore the relationship between health and plant selection to target plants and to isolate bioactive compounds. Several bioactive extracts of plant species eaten by chimpanzees were investigated, some of them leading to novel molecules. Bioguided fractionation of the leaves' extract of *Trichilia rubescens* (Meliaceae) provided two new antiplasmodial limonoids, with similar levels of *in vitro* inhibitory activity as that of chloroquine (Krief *et al.*, 2004). Additionally, we showed that soil when ingested almost simultaneously with *T. rubescens* leaves, increases the bioactivities of *T. rubescens*, suggesting that the feeding behaviour of apes may be more complex than simple addition of food items (Klein *et al.*, 2008). From *Albizia grandibracteata* (Fabaceae) bark and leaves, 4 novel oleanane-type triterpene saponins with antitumor and anthelminthic properties were determined (Krief *et al.*, 2005c). Two other species eaten by chimpanzees (*Warburgia ugandensis* and *Markhamia platycalyx*) have been studied and novel compounds were isolated from active extracts (Lacroix *et al.*, 2009; Xu *et al.*, 2009). Ten novel cycloartanes triterpenoids from *M. platycalyx* (Bignoniaceae) exhibiting antitrypanosomal activities were found. In addition, there is a large overlap between the ingested plant parts by chimpanzees and those used in traditional medicine (Krief *et al.*, 2005a).

Which are the diseases affecting wild chimpanzees?

Diseases in natural populations of apes remain understudied. However their devastating effects on apes population have been highlighted (Walsh *et al.*, 2003; Leendertz *et al.*, 2004; 2006a; 2006b) and recently human diseases transmission sometimes due to spatial proximity was recently recognised as a major threat for their survival (Woodford *et al.*, 2002, Kondgen *et al.*, 2008; Kaur *et al.*, 2008, Boesch, 2008, Williams *et al.*, 2008).

We have been conducting a long-term monitoring of Kanyawara chimpanzees' health, focusing our research on parasites. Since we started our work in Kibale National Park (NP), the intestinal parasite loads of Kanyawara chimpanzees were evaluated (Krief *et al.*, 2003, 2005b, 2010a). This kind of investigation revealed that parasitic burdens were low even if nearly all the individuals were infected. These results suggested a potential regulation of intestinal parasitism (Krief, 2004). The disease caused by the nodular worm *Oesophagostomum bifurcum* can be lethal for humans (Storey *et al.*, 2000a; Storey *et al.*, 2000b, Storey *et al.*, 2001, Storey *et al.*, 2002) and thus it is of major human health significance in certain African regions. Though prevalence of *Oesophagostomum* eggs is high in faecal samples of wild chimpanzees (File *et al.*. 1976; Hasegawa *et al.*, 1983; Huffman *et al.*, 1997), no symptoms had been recorded in chimpanzees. We recently described 6 cases of multinodular oesophagostomosis in ex-captive chimpanzees and in gorillas raised in sanctuaries (Krief *et al.*, 2008). Among other factors, that the access and the use of rough leaves and medicinal plants by orphaned apes' is reduced may explain this difference. There are still gaps in the understanding of the epidemiology of Oesophagostomosis including the role of non-human primates as reservoirs of the infection. *O. stephanostomum* was so far the only species previously found in chimpanzees. We examined 311 stool samples of chimpanzees from Kibale NP and we detected for the first time *O. bifurcum* by PCR amplification as well as a higher parasite load in high ranking males (Krief *et al.*, 2010a).

Malaria is a major parasitic infection, infecting and killing several million people each year. Chimpanzees and gorillas are known to harbour malaria parasites (genus *Plasmodium*) similar to those that infect humans. However, few studies of parasites in African apes have been conducted to date and few symptoms that might be attributed to malaria were recorded in apes. Recently, Olomo *et al.*. (2009) discovered a new malaria agent infecting chimpanzees in Central Africa, named *Plasmodium gaboni*, a close relative of the most pathogenic human agent *P. falciparum*. Using PCR amplification, we detected *Plasmodium* parasites in blood samples from 18 of 91 individuals of the genus *Pan*, including six chimpanzees (three *Pan troglodytes troglodytes*, three *Pan t. schweinfurthii*) and twelve bonobos (*Pan paniscus*). In chimpanzees, we identified two new parasite species closely related to *P. falciparum*, the most dangerous of the parasites in humans. We also found that bonobos harbour malaria parasites including *P. falciparum* (Krief *et al.*, 2010 a). The 3 sampled chimpanzees from Kibale NP harboured complex mixed strain/species infections suggesting that prevalence of infections under natural conditions of transmission is high (Krief *et al.*, 2010b). Our data indicate that chimpanzees and bonobos can maintain malaria parasites, to which humans are susceptible.

How do apes select medicinal plants?

Except for an experimental study targeted on rough leaves supporting an opportunistic original acquisition later passed as a tradition (Huffman and Hirata, 2004), studies investigate preferences of primates related to items having a nutritional value, not towards medicinal plants. Food neophobia, the reluctance to eat unfamiliar food, shows heritable variation in humans (Knaapila *et al.*, 2007) and was widely investigated in captive monkeys (Visalberghi and Addessi, 2000; Addessi and Visalberghi, 2001; Visalberghi *et al.*, 2003) to explain diet acquisition and preferences. Studies on food choices in captive apes have been conducted (Visalberghi *et al.*, 2002; Ueno, 2005; Wobber *et al.*, 2008) but are still rare. However, it seems that mothers rarely actively interfere with infant's activity and mothers have been rarely reported discarding food from infant mouth or hand (Nishida *et al.*, 1983; Goodall, 1986). Rather, infants show referencing behaviour to mothers when encountering a novel food (Ueno, 2005). We investigated in captive orangutans, individual and social learning involved in the discovery and ingestion of new items. We presented novel aromatic plants – 11 fresh plants and 4 infused plants – to 4 captive weaned Bornean orangutans, both under isolated and group conditions, and recorded their behaviour and interactions between group members. All animals tasted by nibbling or ingested most of the plants presented. Regardless of the experimental condition, individual responses did not vary visibly across the sessions, despite numerous close observations, and food transfers between individuals were observed. Our results suggest that a low level of neophobia and a strong propensity to look to conspecifics for information allow Bornean orangutans to expand their diet after weaning. Our results also provide some evidence that olfaction is a key sense in determining food edibility based on previous experience.

Discussion and perspectives

Tropical forests are being threatened by accelerating rate of forest conversion and degradation. They contain however 50 to 90% of the animal and vegetal species and remain the main source for medicinal products. Of all the primates, 90% live in tropical forests and one in five is endangered or critically endangered. The unique habitat of six species of great apes (2 species of chimpanzees, 2 species of gorillas, 2 species of orangutans) is tropical forest. In the framework of our partnership with Ugandan institutions, we aim at implementing the knowledge on phytochemistry and biodiversity of Ugandan plants using chimpanzees as 'guides'. Studying and preserving the interactions between humans, animals and flora is of major interest for the human health and the planet welfare in the future.

It is the challenge of the seventh species of great apes, present worldwide and threatening the others, human beings, to save their closest parents, umbrella and keystone species in tropical forests.

References

Addessi E, Visalberghi E (2001) Social facilitation of eating novel food in tufted capuchin monkeys (*Cebus apella*): Input provided by group members and responses affected in the observer. Anim Cognition 4:297-303.

Baker M (1996) Fur Rubbing: Use of Medicinal Plants by Capucin Monkeys (*Cebus capucinus*), Am J Primatology 38:263-270.

Birkinshaw CR (1999) Use of Millipedes by Black Lemurs to Anoint their Bodies. Folia Primatologica 70:170–171.

Bjone SJ, Brown WY, Price IR (2007) Grass eating patterns in the domestic dog, *Canis familiaris*. Recent Adv Anim Nutr in Australia 16:45-49.

Bjone SJ, Brown WY, Price IR (2009) Maternal influence on grass-eating behavior in puppies. J Vet Behavior 4:97-98.

Boesch C (2008) Why do chimpanzees die in the forest? The challenges of understanding and controlling for wild ape health. Am J Primatology 70:722-726.

Chapuisat M, Oppliger A, Magliano P, Christe P (2007) Wood ants use resin to protect themselves against pathogens. Proc Roayl Soc of London, Series B, 274:2013-2017.

Christe P, Oppliger A, Bancalà F, Castella G, Chapuisat M (2003) Evidence for collective medication in ants. Ecology Letters 6:19-22.

Clark L, Masson JR (1985) Use of Nest Material as Insecticidal and Anti-Pathogenic Agents by the European Starling. Oecologia 67:169-176.

Clark L, Masson JR (1988) Effect of Biologically Active Plants Used as Nest Material and the Derived Benefits to Starling Nestlings. Oecologia 77:174-780.

Clayton DH (1999) Feather-Busting Bacteria. The Auk 116:302-304.

File SK, Mc Grew WC, Tutin CEG (1976) The intestinal parasites of a community of feral chimpanzees, *Pan troglodytes schweinfurthii*. J Parasitol 62:259-261.

Gompper ME, Hoylman AM (1993) Grooming with Trattinickia Resin: Possible Pharmaceutical Plant Use by Coatis in Panama. J Tropical Ecology 9:533-540.

Goodall J (1986) The Chimpanzes of Goombe: Patterns of behavior. Cambridge: Harvard University Press. Pp: 673

Hasegawa H, Kano T, Mulavwa M (1983) A parasitological survey on the feces of Pygmy chimpanzees, *Pan paniscus*, at Wamba, Zaire. Primates 24:419-423.

Hoppe-Dominik B (1988) Grass-eating leopards: Wolves turned into sheep? Naturwissenschaften 75: 49-50; DOI: 10.1007/BF00367444.

Huffman MA, Gotoh S, Turner L, Yoshida K (1997) Seasonal trends in intestinal nematode infection and medicinal plant use among chimpanzees in the Mahale Mountains, Tanzania. Primates 38:111-125.

Huffman MA, Hirata S (2004) An experimental study of leaf swallowing in captive chimpanzees- insights into the origin of a self-medicative behavior and the role of social learning. Primates 45: 113-118.

Huffman MA, Seifu M (1989) Observations of illness and consumption of a possibly medicinal plant Vernonia amygdalina (Del.), by a wild chimpanzee in the Mahale Mountains National Park, Tanzania. Primates 30:51-63.

Huffman MA, Wrangham RW (1994) Diversity of medicinal plants use by chimpanzees in the wild. In *Chimpanzee cultures*, RW Wrangham, WC McGrew, FB de Wall, PG Heltne (Eds). Harvard University Press, Mass. Pp 129-148.

Kaur T. Singh J, Tong S, Humphrey C, Clevenger D, Tan W, Szekely B, Wang Y, Li Y, Alex Muse E, Kiyono M, Hanamura S, Inoue E, Nakamura M, Huffman MA, Jiang B, Nishida T (2008) Descriptive epidemiology of fatal respiratory outbreaks and detection of a human-related metapneumovirus in wild chimpanzees (*Pan troglodytes*) at Mahale Mountains National Park, Western Tanzania. Am J Primatology 70:755-765.

Klein N, Fröhlich F, Krief S (2008) Geophagy: soil consumption enhances the bioactivities of plants eaten by chimpanzees. Naturwissenschaften 95:325-331.

Knaapila H, Tuorila K, Silventoinen K, Keskitalo M, Kallela M, Wessman L, Peltonen LF, Cherkas T, Spector TD, Perola M (2007) Food neophobia shows heritable variation in humans. Phys Behavior 91:573-578.

Köndgen S, Kühl H, N'Goran PK, Walsh PD, Schenk S, Ernst N, Biek R, Formenty P, Matz-Rensing K, Schweiger B, Junglen S, Ellerbrok H, Nitsche A, Briese T, Lipkin WI, Pauli G, Boesch C, Leendertz FH (2008) Pandemic human viruses cause decline of endangered great apes. Curr Biol 18:260-264.

Krief S (2004). Effets prophylactiques et thérapeutiques de plantes ingérées par les chimpanzés: la notion d'« automédication » chez les chimpanzés. Primatologie 6:171-191.

Krief S, Bories C, Hladik CM (2003) Résultats des examens parasitologiques de selles pratiqués sur une population de chimpanzés sauvages (*Pan troglodytes schweinfurthii*) d'Ouganda. Bull Soc Pathologie Exotique 96:80-82

Krief S, Escalante A, Pacheco MA, Mugisha L, André C, Halbwax M, Fischer A, Krief JM, Kasenene J, Crandfield M, Cornejo O, Chavatte JM, Lin C, Letourneur F, Gruner AC, McCutchan T, Rénia L, Snounou G (2010b) On the diversity of malaria parasites in African Apes and the origin of *Plasmodium falciparum* from bonobos. PLOS PathogenS, 6: e1000765.

Krief S, Hladik CM, Haxaire C (2005a) Ethnomedicinal and bioactive properties of plants ingested by wild chimpanzees in Uganda. J Ethnopharmacology 101:1-15.

Krief S, Huffman M, Sévenet T, Guillot J, Bories C, Hladik CM, Wrangham RW (2005b) Noninvasive monitoring of the health of *Pan troglodytes schweinfurthii* in the Kibale National Park, Uganda. Int J Primatology 26:467-490.

Krief S, Martin MT, Grellier P, Kasenene J, Sévenet T (2004) Novel antimalarial compounds isolated after the survey of self-medicative behavior of wild chimpanzees in Uganda. Antimicrobial Agents and Chemotherapy 48:3196-3199.

Krief S, Thoison O, Sévenet T, Wrangham R, Lavaud C (2005c) Triterpenoid saponin anthranilates from *Albizia grandibracteata* leaves ingested by Primates in Uganda. J Natural Products 68: 897-903.

Krief S, Vermeulen B, Lafosse S, Kasenene JM, Nieguitsila A, Berthelemy M, L'Hostis M, Bain O, Guillot J (2010a) Nodular worm infection in wild chimpanzees in Western Uganda: a risk for human health? PLOS Neglected Tropical Diseases 4:e630.

Lacroix D, Prado S, Deville A, Krief S, Dumontet V, Kasenene J, Mouray E, Bories C, Bodo B (2009) Hydroperoxy-cycloartane triterpenoids from the leaves of *Markhamia lutea*, a plant ingested by wild chimpanzees. Phytochemistry 70:1239-1245.

Leendertz FH, Junglen S, Boesch C, Formenty P, Couacy-Hymann E, Courgnaud V, Pauli G, Ellerbrok E (2004) High Variety of Different Simian T-Cell Leukemia Virus Type 1 Strains in Chimpanzees (*Pan troglodytes verus*) of the Taï National Park, Côte d'Ivoire. J Virology 78:4352-4356.

Leendertz FH, Pauli G, Maetz-Rensing K, Boardman W, Nunn C, Ellerbrok H, Jensen SA, Junglen S, Boesch C (2006a) Pathogens as drivers of population declines: The importance of systematic monitoring in great apes and other threatened mammals. Biol Conserv 131:325-337.

Leendertz FH, Yumlu S, Pauli G, Boesch C, Couacy-Hymann E, Vigilant L, Junglen S, Schenk S, Ellerbrok H (2006b) A new Bacillus anthracis kills wild chimpanzees and gorilla in West and Central Africa. PLOS Pathogens 2:e8.

Lefèvre T, Oliver L, Hunter MD, De Roode JC (2010) Evidence for trans-generational medication in nature. Ecology Letters 13:1485-1493. doi: 10.1111/j.1461-0248.2010.01537.

McKenzie SJ, Brown WY, Price IR (2010) Reduction in grass eating behaviours in the domestic dog, *Canis familiaris*, in response to a mild gastrointestinal disturbance. Appl Anim Behav Sci 123:51-55.

Nishida T, Wrangham RW, Goodall J, Uehara S (1983) Local differences in plant feeding habits of chimpanzees between the Mahale Mountains and Gombe National Park, Tanzania. J Human Evolution 12:467-480.

Ollomo B, Durand P, Prugnolle F, Douzery E, Arnathau C, Nkoghe D, Leroy E, Renaud F (2009) A New Malaria Agent in African Hominids. PLOS Pathogen 5:e1000446.

Petit C, Hossaert-McKey M, Perret P, Blondel J, Lambrechts MM (2002) Blue Tits Selected Plants and Olfaction to Maintain an Aromatic Environment for Nestlings. Ecology Letters 5:585-589.

Singer MS, Mace KC, Bernays EA (2009) Self-medication as adaptive plasticity: increased ingestion of plant toxins by parasitized caterpillars. PLOS ONE 4:e4796.

Storey PA, Faile G, Hewitt E, Yelifari L, Polderman AM, Magnussen P (2000b) Clinical epidemiology and classification of human oesophagotomiasis. Royal Soc Trop Med 94:177-182.

Storey PA, Anemana S, van Oostayen JA, Magnussen P, Polderman AM (2000a) Ultrasound diagnosis of oesophagostomiasis. Br J Radiol 73:328-332.

Storey PA, Spannbrucker N. Agongo EA, Van Lieshout L, Zeim JP, Magnussen P, Polderman AM, Doehring E (2002) Intraobserver and interobserver variation of ultrasound diagnosis of *Oesophagostomum bifurcum* colon lesions. Am J Trop Hyg 67:680-683.

Storey PA, Steenhard NR, Van Lieshout L, Anemana S, Magnussen P, Polderman AM (2001) Natural progression of *Oesophagostomum bifurcum* pathology and infection in rural community of northern Ghana. Royal Soc Trop Med 95:295-299.

Sueda KLC, Hart BL, Cliff KD (2008) Characterisation of plant eating in dogs. Appl Anim Behav Sci 111:120-132.

Termonia A, Pasteels JM, Windsor DM, Milinkovitch MC (2002) Dual chemical sequestration: a key mechanism in transitions among ecological specialization. Proc Royal Soc London, Series B 269:1–6.

Ueno A (2005) Development of co-feeding behavior in young wild Japanese macaques (*Macaca fuscata*). Infant Behavior Development 28:481-491.

Visalberghi E, Myowa Yamakoshi M, Hirata S, Matsuzawa T (2002) Responses to novel foods in captive chimpanzees. Zoo Biol 21:539-548.

Visalberghi E, Adessi E (2000) Seeing group members eating a familiar food enhances the acceptance of novel foods in capuchin monkeys. Anim Behavior 60:69-76.

Visalberghi E, Janson CH, Agostini I (2003) Response toward novel foods and novel objects in wild *Cebus apella*. Int J Primatology 24:653-675.

Walsh CF *et al.* (2003) Catastrophic Ape decline in western equatorial Africa. Nature 422:611-614.

Williams DE (2008). Self-medication in horses PhD thesis, Colorado State Univ, USA.

Williams JM, Lonsdorf EV, Wilson ML, Schumacher-Stankey J, Goodall J, Pusey AE (2008) Causes of death in the Kasekela chimpanzees of Gombe National Park, Tanzania. Am J Primatology 70:766-777.

Wobber V, Hare B, Wrangham RW. (2008) Great apes prefer cooked food. J Human Evolution 55:340-348.

Woodford MH, Butynski TM, Karesh WB (2002) Habituating the great apes: the disease risks. Oryx 36:153-160.

Wrangham RW, Nishida T (1983) *Aspilia* spp. leaves: a puzzle in the feeding behavior of wild chimpanzees. Primates 24:276-282.

Xu M. Litaudon M, Krief S, Martin MT, Kasenene J, Kiremire B, Dumontet V, Guéritte F (2009) Ugandenial A, a new drimane-type sesquiterpenoid from *Warburgia ugandensis*. Molecules 14:3844-3850.

Feed supplements to maintain performance and health

Kenneth Harrington McKeever
Equine Science Center, Rutgers, the State University of New Jersey, Dept.
Animal Science, 84 Lipman Drive, New Brunswick, NJ 08901, USA;
mckeever@aesop.rutgers.edu

Recent reports in the literature confirm the links between exercise, inflammation, immune system response and the use of food components and nutraceuticals to modulate these responses (Franke *et al.*, 2005). To that end, recent work conducted at Rutgers examined the anti-inflammatory effects of a number of food extracts. In vitro studies demonstrated efficacy in cell culture and a rodent model demonstrated efficacy in reducing experimentally induced-inflammation model (Franke *et al.*, 2005). Follow up studies focused on the most promising extracts with the horse utilized as an intermediate animal model (Franke *et al.*, 2005). Those studies were funded by the US Department of Defense with the rationale that food extracts with anti-inflammatory properties could replace or reduce the use of non-steroidal anti-inflammatory drugs (NSAIDS) for the reduction of delayed onset muscle soreness in humans.

Equine athletes like their human counterparts suffer from challenges to the immune system and inflammation related to exercise. Published information and current research have sought new anti-inflammatory medications to replace phenylbutazone the most common NSAID given to horses. Work currently being conducted at several feed supplement and pharmaceutical companies is examining the effects of food extracts cytokines and other markers of inflammation. The endocrine and immune function responses to the challenges of exercise and aging are very similar in horses and humans. Much of the current exploration of the use of nutraceuticals in the equine athlete is centered on the immune enhancing and anti-inflammatory properties of those products. We have recently published several studies that have examined the effects of various pharmaceutical and nutraceutical interventions on exercise capacity. Treadmill tests that have been used have included incremental exercise tests to measure aerobic and physiological markers of performance, simulated race tests and high intensity exercise tests, and endurance exercise tests. The present paper present a series of abstracts that have been published from studies that were used to screen the safety, pharmacokinetics, and efficacy, of functional food extracts.

The general goal of the research presented was to determine if the chosen extracts would alter markers of performance as well as cytokine markers of post-exertion inflammation and muscle damage in an animal model, the horse. The extracts examined were chosen from more than a dozen screened in various in vitro and rodent models for their ability to alter markers of inflammation. The horse was chosen as an animal model because of its ability to perform exercise, its physiological similarities to humans, the ease of administration of extracts, and the ability to collect blood and muscle samples to obtain both pharmacokinetic and pharmacodynamic information. Pharmacokinetic and pharmacodynamic information from these experiments answer the key questions that should be asked when considering if a supplement should be used in the care of an equine athlete (McKeever, 2005).

Study 1: Effect of ephedra on thermoregulation and exercise performance[1]

Norton RP, Lehnhard RA, Kearns CF, McKeever KH. Equine Science Center, Rutgers the State University of New Jersey and the Department of Kinesiology, University of Maine.

The dietary supplement ephedra is a potent sympathomimetic that was banned by the US Food and Drug Administration in 2006 because of its deleterious effects on cardiovascular function and thermoregulation during exercise. Unfortunately, extracts of ephedra can still be obtained via the internet and are in use worldwide. The horse is the only athletic species other than humans that sweats to thermoregulate and it controls cardiovascular function in a similar fashion. The

---

[1] Ephedra-induced alterations in cardiovascular function and thermoregulation during acute exercise in horses. Med Sci Sport Exerc, submitted for review, September, 2011).

purpose of this study was to use the horse to examine the acute effects of ephedra (Ma Huang) to investigate on markers of performance as well as effects on cardiovascular function and thermoregulation during acute exercise. Six Standardbred mares ($\sim$450 kg; 6-12 yrs of age) were used in a crossover design consisting of an ephedra (Ma Huang containing 8% ephedra alkaloid) and control (applesauce) group. All horses performed an incremental exercise test (GXT) at a 6% fixed grade to measure maximal oxygen uptake (VO_{2max}), run time, velocity at VO_{2max}, maximal velocity, recovery time, hematocrit, total plasma protein concentration, heart rate, right ventricular pressure (RVP), pulmonary arterial pressure (PAP), rectal temperature and recovery. All measurements were recorded at rest, during exercise and post 2 and 5 minute recovery. There was a significant difference ($P<0.05$) in pre-exercise hematocrit but not in any other hematocrit or plasma protein sampling intervals. VO_2 was significantly higher for the ephedra group before exercise, at each step of the graded exercise test (GXT), at VO_{2max}, and during recovery compared to the control group. Recovery time was significantly different, but run time was not ($P>0.05$). Heart rate was significantly elevated at 2 and 5 min. recovery in horses administered ephedra. Significant differences were observed for RVP and PAP and rectal temperature during recovery. Recovery score (sweating response, respiration rate, behavior) was altered ($P<0.05$) by ephedra administration. This data suggests an increase in energy expenditure and thermogenesis when horses consume ephedra. However, markers of performance (run time, velocity at VO_{2max}, and maximal velocity completed) were not altered by ephedra administration.

Study 2: Effect of orange peel extract and black tea on marker s of performance and inflammation[2]

Streltsova JM, McKeever KH, Lihurt NR, Manso HC, Gordon ME, Horohov D, Rosen R, Franke W. Equine Science Center, Center for Advanced Food Technology, and the Department of Food Science, Rutgers the State University of New Jersey and the Maxwell H Gluck Equine Research Center, University of Kentucky.

[2] Abstract previously published and used with permission: Effect of orange peel and black tea extracts on markers of performance and cytokine markers of inflammation in horses. Eq Comp Exerc Physiol 3:121-130, 2006).

This study tested the hypothesis that orange peel (O) and decaffeinated black tea (T) extracts would alter markers of exercise performance as well as exercise-induced mRNA expression for the inflammatory cytokines IL-6, TNF-α and IFN-γ. Nine healthy, unfit Standardbred mares (age: $10+4$ yrs, ~ 450 kg) were assigned to 3 treatment groups in a randomized crossover design where each horse was administered one of the following; placebo (O; 2 L water), black tea extract in water (T; 2 L), or orange peel extract in water (W; 2 L), via a nasogastric tube. One hour later the horses completed an incremental graded exercise test (GXT) on a treadmill at a fixed 6% grade with measurements and blood samples obtained at rest, at the end of each 1 min. step of the GXT and at 2 and 5 min. post GXT. An additional set of blood samples for PCR measurement of mRNA were obtained before exercise and at 5 min, 30 min., and 1, 2, 4, and 24 hr. post-GXT. The GXTs were conducted between 07:00 and 12:00 no less than 7 d apart. There were no differences ($P>0.05$) in VO_{2max}, respiratory exchange ratio, run time, velocity at VO_{2max}, core body temperature, hematocrit, creatine kinase, plasma lactate concentrations, HR, right ventricular pressure, or pulmonary artery pressure across treatments. A major finding was that orange peel extract significantly reduced post-exercise VO_2 recovery time ($W=112+7$, $O=86+6$, $T=120+11$ s). There was a significant difference in plasma total protein concentration (TP) in the O runs compared to water and T. TNF-α mRNA expression was lower in the T runs compared to water and O trials. IFN-γ mRNA expression levels appeared to be lower in both the T and O extract runs compared to the water trials. The mRNA expression of IL-6 was unaltered across treatment groups. These data suggest that orange peel and black tea extracts may modulate the cytokine responses to intense exercise. Orange peel extract reduced post-exercise recovery time and may potentially enhance the ability of horses to perform subsequent bouts of high intensity exercise.

Study 3: Effect of cranberry and ginger extracts on markers of performance and inflammation[3]

Liburt NR, K.H. McKeever KH, Streltsova JM, Franke WC, Gordon ME, Manso Filho HC, Horohov DW, Rosen RT, Ho CT, Singh AP, Vorsa N. Equine Science Center, Center for Advanced Food Technology, Department of Food Science, and the Philip E Marucci Center for Blueberry and Cranberry Research and Extension, Rutgers the State University of New Jersey and the Maxwell H Gluck Equine Research Center, University of Kentucky.

This study hypothesized that ginger (*Zingiber officinale*) and cranberry (*Vaccinium macrocarpon*) extracts would alter the physiological response to exercise as well as markers of muscle damage, and mRNA expression for the inflammatory cytokines tumor necrosis factor-alpha (TNF-α), interferon-gamma (IFN-γ) and interleukin-6 (IL-6) after an exhaustive bout of exercise in horses. Nine unfit Standardbred mares (age 10 ± 4 yrs, ~450 kg) completed 3 graded exercise tests (GXT) in a crossover design where they were assigned to the initial order of treatment in a randomized fashion. The GXTs were conducted between 07:00 and 12:00, 7 days apart. Mares received either water (2 l), cranberry (~30 g in 2 l water) or ginger (~30 g in 2 l water) extract 1 h prior to testing. Blood samples were taken prior to dosing (pre-ex), at the end of each step of the GXT, end of exercise, 2, 5 and 30 min, 1, 2, 4 and 24 h post-GXT. Plasma total protein concentration (TP) and hematocrit (HCT) were analyzed immediately following the tests. Analysis of creatine kinase (CK) and aspartate aminotransferase (AST) were done commercially. There was no effect of treatment ($P>0.05$) on VO$_{2max}$, run-time to fatigue, core temperature, TP or HCT. CK was substantially elevated ($P<0.05$) in the ginger group at 4 h post-GXT. All CK levels returned to baseline 24 h post-GXT. No change ($P>0.05$) was noted in AST. A slight increase ($P<0.05$) in CK was seen in all groups at 2 h post-GXT. The cranberry group had significantly lower TNF-α mRNA expression compared to control and ginger. Ginger appeared to influence ($P<0.05$) the upregulation and expression of IFN-γ mRNA at 30 min-post GXT, but, more strikingly, significantly decreased recovery time defined as the time for VO$_2$ to recover from the peak

---

[3] Abstract previously published and used with permission: Effects of cranberry and ginger on the physiological response to exercise and markers of inflammation following acute exercise in horses. Comp Exerc Physiol 6:157-169, 2009).

observed at fatigue to a post-exercise plateau (ginger $= 101 \pm 3$ s, water $= 130 \pm 14$ s, cranberry $= 131 \pm 16$ s). No effect of treatment or exercise ($P > 0.05$) was seen on IL-6 mRNA expression. Results suggest that cranberry extract blunts the upregulation and expression of TNF-α mRNA, while ginger extract reduces cardiovascular recovery time in horses completing a short, exhaustive bout of exercise.

Study 4: Uptake and distribution of cranberry flavanols into muscle in horses

Malone S, McKeever KH, Liburt NL, Franke WC, Singh A, Vorsa N. Equine Science Center, Center for Advanced Food Technology, Department of Food Science, Philip E Marucci Center for Blueberry and Cranberry Research and Extension, Rutgers the State University of New Jersey.

In our first 2005 study ethyl acetate cranberry extract was administered via NG tube to 1 horse. Flavanols were detected in plasma and urine within 15 min; however, the study did not measure in muscle the key end tissue. For the 2008 study cranberry 90 MX powder was administered to 3 horses in a crossover study (Table 1). Horses were administered either 0, 200, or 400 g of cranberry in 2 liters water via NG tube. Plasma, muscle, urine samples were collected before administration and at 0.5, 1, 2, 4, 6, 12, and 24 hrs post-administration.

Table 1. The peak time and peak concentration (μg/g) in horse muscle for each of the flavonols in the low dose (LD, 200 mg) and high dose (HD, 400 mg) of the cranberry powder. The data is expressed at the means ± SE mean (n = 3). An asterisk (*) indicates the mean peak concentration was significantly different from the pre-dosing control.

Flavanol	Time to peak (hrs)		Peak concentration		24 hr concentration	
	LD	HD	LD	HD	LD	HD
Q-3 Galactoside	4	1	2.31±2.14	1.22±0.83*	0	0.03±0.03
Q-3 Arabinofuranoside	4	1	0.12±0.07*	0.07±0.04*	0	0
Q-3 Rhamnoside	4	1	0.54±0.51	0.23±0.20	0	0.02±0.02
M-3 Galactoside	4	1	0.78±0.76	0.37±0.21*	0	0
Q-3 Arabinopyranoside	4	16	0.19±0.17*	0.05±0.05	0.02±0.02	0
Quercetin	4	4	1.93±1.83*	5.25±5.19*	0.10±0.04	0.16±0.13

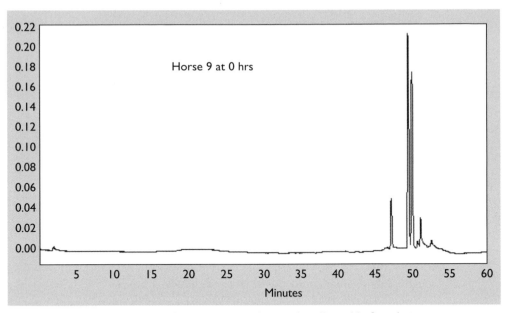

Figure 1. HPLC chromatograms from horse muscle sample collected before dosing.

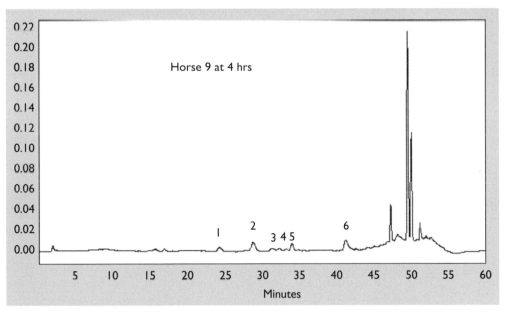

Figure 2. HPLC chromatograms from a horse muscle sample taken from the horse in Figure 1, but at 4 hrs post-dosing. The flavonols associated with the peaks are identified as: (1) M-3 Galactoside; (2) Quercetin-3 Galactoside; (3) Quercetin-3 Arabinopyranoside; (4) Quercetin-3 Arabinofuranoside; (5) Quercetin-3 Rhamnoside, and (6) Quercetin.

Each trial was performed with one month between each rounds to allow complete recovery from the multiple biopsies. Figure 1 demonstrates the HPLC readout for a muscle sample taken before cranberry extract administration (control) and Figure 2 demonstrates the pattern of peaks for the key flavanols that appeared in a muscle sample collected 4 hours after administration.

The major conclusion of this pilot study was that there was a rapid uptake and clearance of the key flavanols found in cranberry extract. Some flavanols were detected in plasma in early samples, a minimal amount detected in urine, and substantial amount in muscle. These observations were similar to rat studies where flavanols were cleared rapidly from plasma with large amounts measured in the tissues (liver and kidneys). It was also concluded that quercetin was the major flavonol present in horse muscle and blood. Quercetin has been shown to be the most active anti-inflammatory flavanol in many functional foods.

Study 5: Exercise-induced increases in inflammatory cytokines in muscle and blood[4]

Liburt NR, Horohov DW, Betancourt A, Adams AA, Franke WC, McKeever KH. Equine Science Center and the Center for Advanced Food Technology, Rutgers the State University of New Jersey and the Maxwell H Gluck Equine Research Center, University of Kentucky.

Studies have demonstrated increases in mRNA expression for inflammatory cytokines following exercise in horses and have suggested those markers of inflammation may play a role in delayed onset muscle soreness. However, measurement of mRNA expression in white blood cells is an indirect method. No studies to date have documented the cytokine response to exercise directly in muscle. This study tested the hypothesis that exercise increases cytokine markers of inflammation in blood and muscle. Blood and muscle biopsies were obtained from four healthy, unfit Standard bred mares ($\sim$ 500 kg). The randomized crossover experiment was performed with the investigators blind to the treatment. Each horse underwent either

---

[4] Abstract previously published and used with permission: Exercise-induced increases in cytokine markers of inflammation in muscle and blood in horses. Eq Vet J Suppl 38:280-288, 2010).

incremental exercise test (GXT) or standing parallel control with one month between trials. During the GXT horses ran on a treadmill (1 m/s increases each min until fatigue, 6% grade). Blood and muscle biopsies were obtained 30 min before, immediately after, and at 0.5, 1, 2, 6, and 24 hrs post-GXT or at matched time points during parallel control trials. Samples were analyzed using real time-PCR for measurement of mRNA expression of interferon-gamma (IFN-γ), tumor necrosis factor-alpha (TNF-α), interleukin-6 (IL-6), and interleukin-1 (IL-1). Data were analyzed using t-tests with the null hypothesis rejected when $P < 0.10$. There were no changes ($P > 0.10$) in IL-1, IL-6, IFN-γ, or TNF-α during control. Exercise induced significant increases in IFN-γ, IL1, and TNF-α in blood and significant increases in IFN-γ, IL-6, and TNF-α in muscle. There were no significant changes in mRNA expression of IL-1 in muscle or IL-6 in blood following the GXT. Cytokine markers of inflammation all returned to pre-GXT levels by 24 hrs post-GXT.

Study 6: Effects of cranberry extracts on the glucose and insulin response to intense exercise in horses

Roos J, McKeever KH, Liburt NL, Franke WC, Vorsa N. Rutgers the State University of New Jersey.

Previous studies have demonstrated that ginger (*Zingiber officinale*) and cranberry (*Vaccinium macrocarpon*) extracts alter markers of performance and mRNA expression for inflammatory cytokines after an exhaustive bout of exercise in horses. Those cytokines may alter the insulin response to acute intense exercise. Therefore, nine unfit Standard bred mares (age 10 ± 4 yrs, ~450 kg) were used to test the hypothesis that ginger and cranberry would alter the insulin response after intense exertion. Each mare completed 3 graded exercise tests (GXTs) in a randomized crossover design with the investigators blind to the treatment. The tests were conducted between 07:00 and 12:00 no less than 7 d apart. Mares received either water (2 l), cranberry (~30 g in 2 l water), or ginger (~30 g in 2 l water) extract 1 h prior to testing. Blood samples were taken prior to dosing (about -1 hr to exercise), immediately after exercise (0 hr) and at 0.5, 1, 2, 4 and 24 h post-GXT. Plasma insulin concentrations were measured in duplicate using a RIA kit previously validated for use in horses. Data were analyzed using a three-way ANOVA with the null hypothesis rejected when $P < 0.05$.

There was a significant effect of time on plasma insulin concentration with a suppression immediately following GXT followed by a substantial ($P < 0.05$) increase and a return to baseline ($P > 0.05$) between 2 and 4 hrs post-GXT. There was a significant effect of treatment on the insulin response to exercise with lower concentrations at 0.5, 1 and 2 hrs. Glucose concentrations were increased in all 3 groups due to exertion. However, treatment with cranberry extract resulted in significantly lower glucose concentrations compared to water and ginger. These data suggest that food extracts may modulate the glucose and insulin response to exertion.

Study 7: Effects of quercetin on markers of performance and inflammatory cytokines following intense exercise in horses

Baldassari JP, Horohov DW, Betancourt A, Adams AA, Franke WC, McKeever KH. Rutgers, the State University of New Jersey and Maxwell H Gluck Equine Research Center, University of Kentucky.

Quercetin is the major flavanol in cranberries with anti-inflammatory activity. Studies by Davis and coworkers have demonstrated significant effects on mitochondrial function and aerobic capacity with improved performance in rats and humans. Other studies by Neiman and co-workers have demonstrated an effect on blood cytokine markers of inflammation. To date, the published reports have not focused on high intensity exercise. Additional work by Clarkson and co-workers and Mishniak *et al.* (unpublished data) has focused on the pharmacokinetics and pharmacodynamics of quercetin and has documented that quercetin is taken up into the blood stream. Their ongoing work is looking at the performance effects in humans. The protocols above did not determine if quercetin was being taken up into muscle or measure the effects or the effects of quercetin on the cytokine response in muscle. Therefore the first broad objective of the present study was to utilize the horse as an animal model to document that quercetin is taken up by the muscles and to test the hypothesis that quercetin administration would alter markers of performance and cytokine markers of inflammation in blood and muscle. Work by Espy *et al.* (presentation at the AIBS Quercetin workshop, Natick, MA, 2008) has shown that quercetin acts on Glut 2 transporters in intestinal epithelium resulting in a reduction of glucose uptake. This response would be beneficial for individuals with insulin resistance and type II diabetes, but would be detrimental in warfighters performing endurance exercise. Our work using cranberry extracts showed a similar response during recovery, a period when glucose uptake would be very important for glycogen re-synthesis. Both of those experiments only focused on non-exercised individuals or recovery from exercise. The later response involves an increase in glucose uptake and insulin in an effort to get glucose into the muscles for glycogen synthesis during recovery. That response is different to the response during exertion where insulin is suppressed so as to prevent a precipitous decline in blood glucose during exertion. We are unaware of any data documenting the effects of quercetin administration on the glucose and insulin response first during exercise and then secondarily during recovery. Therefore the second objective of the present study was to test the hypothesis that quercetin administration would alter the glucose and insulin responses to exercise and recovery. Six horses were utilized in this experiment with the investigators analyzing the data blind to the treatment given. The studies were conducted in a random crossover experiments with the horses administered either control (2 liters water) or quercetin (10.5 mg/kg, BID, 7 doses) followed by an incremental exercise test as conducted prior published experiments (Streltsova *et al.*, 2006; Liburt *et al.*, 2009). Performance data was collected as per prior experiments and blood samples obtained prior to dosing and prior to exercise and then during each step of the GXT and out to 24 hrs of recovery. Muscle biopsies were obtained before dosing and then before the GXT, and at 2 min, 30 min, 1, 2, 4 and 24 hrs post-GXT. Blood samples were analyzed for hematocrit and plasma glucose, insulin, lactate, electrolytes, and total protein concentrations. Blood and muscle samples were also used to measure mRNA expression for IL-1, IL6, TNF-α, IFN-γ, and granzyme-B (see definition below). There were major effects of exercise but only limited effects of quercetin. The major positive finding was that quercetin administration enhanced the runtime to fatigue and reduced the alactic or fast phase of recovery. This would be beneficial to a warfighter in the field performing repeated high intensity bouts running from point to point. The other major finding was that quercetin administration reduced the granzyme-B response to exertion. Granzyme-B is one of the first cytokines to increase in response to a physiological or immunological challenge. It is an early phase marker used in influenza and vaccine research (Paillot *et al.*, 2007). Finally, quercetin administration did not alter the glucose or insulin response during the GXT or during the recovery period following exertion.

References

Breathnach CC, Sturgill-Wright T, Stiltner JL, Adams AA, Lunn DP, Horohov DW (2006) Foals are interferon gamma-deficient at birth. Vet Immunology Immunopathology 112:199-209.

Franke WC, *et al.* (2005) Combat ration supplements for improved cognitive and physical performance. In: Technical Report submitted to US Army Natick Soldier System Center, Natick, MA for contract no. DAAD 16-03-C-0055.

Franke WC, McKeever KH, Fong D, Huang MT, Rafi M (2009) Combat ration supplements for improved cognitive and physical performance. In: Technical Report submitted to US Army Natick Soldier System Center, Natick, MA for contract no. W911QY-07-C-0007.

Gregoire S, Singh AP, Vorsa N, Koo H (2007) Influence of cranberry phenolics on glucan synthesis by glucosyltransferases and Streptococcus mutans adicogenicity. J Appl Microbiology 103:1960-1968.

Kearns, CF, McKeever KH (2002) Clenbuterol diminishes aerobic performance in horses Med Sci Sport Exerc 34:1976-1985.

Kimura H, Suzui M, Nagao F, Matsumoto K (2001) Highly sensitive determination of plasma cytokines by time-resolved fluoroimmunoassay; effect of bicycle exercise on plasma level of interleukin-1 alpha (IL-1 alpha), tumor necrosis factor alpha (TNF alpha), and interferon gamma (IFN gamma). Analytical Sciences 17:593-597.

Lehnhard RA, Adams AA, Betancourt A, Horohov DW, Liburt NR, Streltsova JM, Franke WC, McKeever KH (2010) Phenylbutazone blocks the cytokine response following a high intensity incremental exercise challenge in horses. Comp Exerc Physiol 7:103-108.

Liburt NR, McKeever KH, Streltsova JM, Franke WC, Gordon ME, Manso Filho HC, Horohov DW, Rosen RT, Ho CT, Singh AP, Vorsa N (2009) Effects of cranberry and ginger on the physiological response to exercise and markers of inflammation following acute exercise in horses. Comp Exerc Physiol 6:157-169.

Liburt NR, Adams A, Betancourt A, Horohov DW, McKeever KH (2010). Exercise-induced increases in cytokine markers of inflammation in muscle and blood in horses. Eq Vet J Suppl 38:280-288.

Livak KJ, Schmittgen TD (2001) Analysis of relative gene expression data using real-time PCR and the $2^{-\Delta\Delta C_T}$ method. Methods 25:402-408.

McKeever KH (2005) Does it Work? Testing the efficacy of feed supplements In: Advances in Equine Nutrition III. Pagan JD (ed). Nottingham University Press, Nottingham UK; Pp 65-68.

McKeever KH, Agans JM, Geiser S, Lorimer P, Maylin GA (2006) Low dose exogenous erythropoietin elicits an ergogenic effect in Standardbred horses. Eq Vet J Suppl 36:233-238.

Moldoveanu AI, Shephard RJ, Shek PN (2001) The cytokine response to physical activity and training. Sports Med 31:115-144.

Paillot R, Kydd JH, MacRaea S, Minke JM, Hannant D, Daly J (2007) New assays to measure equine influenza virus-specific Type 1 immunity in horses. Vaccine 25:7385-7398.

Pedersen BK, Steensberg A, Fischer C, Keller C, Plomgaard P, Febbraio M, Saltin B (2003) Searching for the exercise factor: is IL-6 a candidate? J Muscle Res Cell Motility 24:113-119.

Pedersen BK, Ostrowski K, Rohde T, Bruunsgaard H (1998) The cytokine response to strenuous exercise. Can J Physiol Pharmacol 76:505-511.

Srivastava KC, Mustafa T (1992) Ginger (*Zingiber officinale*) in rheumatism and musculoskeletal disorders. Medical Hypotheses 39:342-348.

Streltsova JM, McKeever KH, Liburt NR, Manso HC, Gordon ME, Horohov DW, Rosen R, Franke WF (2006) Effect of orange peel and black tea extracts on markers of performance and cytokine markers of inflammation in horses. Eq Comp Exerc Physiol 3:121-130.

Suzuki K, Nakaju S, Yamada M, Totsuka M, Sato K, Sugawara K (2002) Systemic inflammatory response to exhaustive exercise. Cytokine Kinetics. Exerc Immunology Rev 8:6-48.

Vassilakopoulos T, Karatza MH, Katsaounou P, Kollintza A, Zakynthinos S, Roussos C (2003) Antioxidants attenuate the plasma cytokine response to exercise in humans. J Appl Physiol 94: 1025-1032.

Vorsa N, Singh A, Shabrova E, Schaich K, Jin H, Quadro L (2007) Bioavailability and tissues distribution of cranberry flavonol glycosides in mice; FASEB J 21:291.

Vvedenskaya IO, Rosen RT, Guido JT, Russell DJ, Mills KA, Vorsa N (2004) Characterization of flavonols in cranberry (*Vaccinium macrocarpon*) powder. J Agric Food Chem 52:188-195.

Weinstock C, Konig D, Harnischmacher R, Keul J, Berg A, Northoff H (1997) Effect of exhaustive exercise stress on the cytokine response. Med Sci Sport Exercise 29:345-354.

Wilson T, Singh AP, Vorsa N, Goettl CD, Kittleson KM, Roe CM, Kastello GM, Ragsdale FR (2008) Human glycemic response and phenolic content of unsweetened cranberry juice. J Medicinal Food 11:46-54.

Youdim KA, McDonald J, Kalt W, Joseph JA (2002) Potential role of dietary flavonoids in reducing microvascular endothelium vulnerability to oxidative and inflammatory insults. J Nutritional Biochem 13:282-288.

Will total mixed rations be the future of horse feeding?

Sarah L. Ralston[1] and Harlan Anderson[2]
[1]Rutgers, the State University of New Jersey, Dept. Animal Science, 84 Lipman Drive, New Brunswick, NJ 08901, USA; Ralston@aesop.rutgers.edu
[2]IdleAcres, 2379 Quimby Ave SW, 55321 Cokato, MN, USA

Introduction

Forage-based total mixed rations (TMR), wherein all the nutritional needs of the animals are met in a single feedstuff, have been used successfully for decades in growing and adult food animals. The advantages to use of TMRs over traditional long stem hay/concentrate rations is the ease of handling, reduced waste, ability to completely control/regulate nutrient intake and, in some regions cost and improved nutrient availability. In addition, in our increasingly non-agricultural societies, horse owners frequently have little knowledge of judging hay quality and adjusting feed intakes of concentrates to accommodate variations in hay nutrient content. The result is frequently over- or underfeeding nutrients. Over feeding nutrients such as nitrogen (protein) and phosphorus are increasingly becoming environmental concerns (Williams et al., 2011; Westendorf et al., 2011). The use of TMRs would allow specific formulation that could meet but not exceed recommended intakes.

The majority of the available 'complete' feeds are usually provided in a pelleted form and are sufficiently dense calorically that they must be offered in very restricted (< 1.5% BW) amounts to avoid obesity. Pelleted complete feeds have also been documented to be associated with a high incidence of gastric ulceration (Flores et al., 2009). Horses can usually consume their total daily allotment of 'complete' pellets in less than 5 or 6 hours, whereas horses allowed free access to feed spend 10 to 12 hours engaged in eating activity. Grain-based concentrates fed in distinct meals, with or without concurrent hay access, result in significant increases in plasma glucose and insulin (Ralston, 1996; Trieber et al., 2005), and may increase the incidence of developmental orthopedic disease (DOD) such as osteochondrosis

(OCD) in predisposed young horses (Ralston, 1996; Pagan *et al.*, 2001), though the association between non structured carbohydrates (NSC) intake and OCD is not 100% (Ralston *et al.*, 2007, 2011). High grain/starch/sugar intakes are also commonly associated with the development of insulin resistance in adult horses (Frank *et al.*, 2010) and aggravation of rhabdomyolysis in horses with polysaccharide storage myopathy (Valberg, 2011).

TMR formulated with grain added

In a series of experiments conducted over the past 7 years we have documented the safety and efficacy of TMRs with or without added grains for use in young horses. In the three initial trials (2004-2006), in October of each year 12 draft cross weanlings were paired by sex and type and fed either TMR cubes (Next Generation™, IdleAcres, Cokato, MN) free choice (TMR, n = 6 per year)) or Nutrena® (Minnetonka, MN) Life Design Youth® (HCY:2004, 2005) or SafeChoice® (HCSC, 2006) to provide 50% of the calories recommended for growth (NRC, 1989) with ad libitum grass/alfalfa mix hay (n = 6 per year) for 6 to 8 weeks. Feed intakes were recorded daily and height and weight were measured weekly. The horses were evaluated visually for the presence of developmental orthopedic disease before and after each trial by an experienced observer blind to the dietary treatments. The studies were repeated for 6-8 weeks each spring in a crossover design. The horses were given a low dose oral dextrose challenge test (0.25 gm dextrose/kg BW, Ralston, 2002) before treatments were initiated and after 6 to 8 weeks on their respective treatments and plasma glucose/insulin responses to consuming equicaloric amounts of the TMR versus concentrate used were also measured. Nutrient content of the rations differed somewhat between years (Table 1). In the first two trials the TMR cubes had 10-15% cracked corn added to the formulation, in the third ground oats were used instead of corn.

Feed efficiency (kg gain/Mcal DE consumed) was higher ($P < 0.05$) in the TMR horses relative to the traditional hay/concentrate horses in all three years and all trials. Growth rates tended ($P < 0.1$) to be slightly higher in the TMR horses and were definitely higher (average of 1.2 kg/day in the draft cross weanlings, 0.8 kg/day in the yearlings) than predicted by NRC (1989) in all three years. The horses voluntarily consumed between 2.5 and 3.0% of their body weight

Table 1. Nutrient content of rations used 2004-2006. Values are on DM basis of feed.

Year/feed	2004 HGY[1]	2004 TMR	2005 HGY[1]	2005 TMR	2006 HGSC[1]	2006 TMR
DE Mcal/kg	2.4	2.2	2.2	2.2	2.6	2.4
% Protein	14.0	18.2	11.0	16.7	14.7	15.6
% NSC	20.0	16.5	20.0	13.0	15.4	15.0
% Ca	0.88	1.47	0.73	1.07	1.00	1.18
% Phos	0.45	0.42	0.35	0.32	0.54	0.32

[1] Based on mean total hay/concentrate consumed per day. Grass/alfalfa mix hay quality in 2004, 2006 was good, 2005 hay was only moderate.

daily as weanlings, in the spring trials voluntary feed intakes tended to decrease to 2.2 to 2.5% BW. In 2005 two weanlings had DOD (flexure deformities and epiphysitis) and were hyperinsulinemic before the treatments were initiated, one was placed on TMR, the other on HGY. The one on TMR resolved, the one on HGY continued to have severe epiphysitis and flexure deformities throughout the study and in the subsequent spring when placed on TMR. In 2006 two horses had DOD (flexure deformities and epiphysitis) that did not resolve on either ration. Plasma glucose responses to the dextrose challenges did not differ between treatments in the first two years but insulin responses tended ($P < 0.1$) to be higher in HGY fed horses, suggesting somewhat reduced insulin sensitivity. In 2006 there were higher ($P < 0.05$) glucose and insulin responses on TMR than HGSC but that was the year the TMR had 10% ground oats added instead of corn and the SafeChoice® pellets had been specifically formulated to have a low glycemic index. Post-prandial glucose and insulin responses to the meal of SafeChoice® were low compared to HCY and the TMR for the first 90 to 120 minutes but then tended to increase and stay higher ($P < 0.05$) than the other treatments for the next 60 to 90 minutes of samples collection (Ralston *et al.*, 2007). The only feed-related adverse event was a recurrent choke in one horse that was fed the pelleted ration which was prevented when the concentrate was soaked in water prior to feeding. The horses were not, however, evaluated for gastric ulceration, though there was no clinical evidence (poor appetite, colic, etc) of ulceration in any of the horses.

The results obtained with the draft crosses were corroborated in a study at another university, using Standardbred yearlings fed either TMR cubes with 25% oats at the rate of 3% BW/day versus equivalent amounts of hay cubes and oats fed separately as discrete meals. The same hay was used in both types of cubes. The horses on the TMR rations again had higher ($P < 0.05$) growth rates (1.69 kg gain/d) and gain to feed ratio (0.9 kg/kg feed intake) than the meal fed animals (0.95 kg gain/day, 0.05 kg gain/kg feed). No gastric ulcerations were found on endoscopic examination in either treatment group (Warren *et al.*, 2011).

TMR formulated without grain

In more recent studies (Ralston *et al.*, 2009) it was hypothesized that grain free forage-based TMR rations could be formulated to meet or exceed all nutrient recommendations for rapid growth when fed free choice and that young horses fed the TMR ration would have comparable or better growth rates and feed efficiency compared to those fed traditional long stem hay/ grain rations. Twelve draft cross weanlings (6 colts and 6 fillies, initially 5 months old) were fed either TMR cubes (Next Generation©, IdleAcres, Cokato, MN) free choice (TMR, n = 6) or hay/concentrate based Nutrena® (Minnetonka, MN) Safe Choice® (SCH, n = 6) to provide 50% of the calories recommended for moderate growth with free choice grass/alfalfa hay (see Table 2 for analyses). This time the TMR ration contained no added grain. Wheat bran (< 5%) was added to increase phosphorus content to recommended concentrations and a trace mineral/vitamins supplement was also included to ensure intakes that met or exceeded the recommendations for growth. All weanlings maintained good general health. No significant DOD was observed in either treatment group. Though the SCH horses started out 2 cm taller than the TMR group (SCH: 137 ± 1.2 cm, TMR: 135 ± 1.3, $P > 0.05$) and 14 kg heavier (SHC: 293 ± 7 kg, TMR: 279 ± 8 kg), there were no differences ($P > 0.1$) between treatment groups with respect to average daily gain, weekly height increase, or feed efficiency despite lower ($P < 0.05$) daily feed intakes by the TMR horses (Table 3). The TMR fed horses actually consumed only 85.5% of the calories recommended for growth relative to the 100% intake of the SCH horses.

Table 2. Grain-free TMR nutrient concentrations versus traditional Hay/concentrate ration[1]. Values are concentration % As Fed based on measured intakes of Hay/Concentrate and TMR cubes.

Nutrient concentrations	SCH	TMR
DE Mcal	2.83	1.97
% Protein	16.9	14.3
%ADF	23.8	24.7
%NSC	13.6	6.4
%Ca	1.3	1.4
%Phos	0.57	0.41
%Mg	0.42	0.26

[1] Weanlings consumed an average of 3.0 kg SCH divided into two feedings and 4.8 kg hay per day versus 6.45 kg TMR cubes.

Table 3. Growth and feed intakes of draft cross weanlings (n=6 per group) fed either SCH (100% of NRC for 0.8 kg/day gain) (SCH) versus ad libitum alfalfa based TMR cubes without added concentrates. Values are means ± SE.

	SCH	TMR
%BW intake	2.75±0.06	2.53±0.06
ADG, kg/day	0.77±0.16	0.85±0.12
Kg gain /Mcal DE	0.04±0.01	0.05±0.01
%NRC[1]	99.8±2.6	85.6±2.7

[1] Percentage of NRC (2007) recommended caloric intake.

In 2009-2010 further trials were conducted using grain-free TMR rations. In 2009-2010 growth rates of 4 yearling mustangs were compared to yearling and weanling draft crosses. The grain-free forage based cubes formula was again used and the TMR was fed free choice. The growth results for the draft crosses were identical to previous years, with the horses voluntarily consuming ~85% of the predicted necessary caloric intake yet sustaining higher growth rates than predicted by NRC (2007) for horses maturing at 650-750 kg. The mustangs consumed 100% of the recommended caloric intake for horses maturing at 450 kg and had the predicted rates of growth.

Again, the horses maintained excellent body condition and there were no adverse effects (i.e. colic, diarrhea, woodchewing, etc.).

The daily cost, based on the commercial price (2009) of the respective feeds (hay: $ 0.41/kg; grain: 0.70/kg, TMR: $ 0.66/kg), was calculated based on actual intakes. It cost an average of $ 4.26/day for the TMR ration versus $ 4.18/day for the SCH. The SCH horses also wasted 0.8 to 1 kg of hay per day, incurring an average loss of about $ 0.30/day in wasted hay that should be added to the daily cost. There was no waste with the cubes. The cost differential between the two rations is further reduced if labor costs are taken into consideration. It was the subjective observation that it took less time to feed the cubes than the hay/grain rations and the bags of cubes were easier to store and handle than the long stem hay bales.

Conclusions

Feeding TMR cubes formulated for growth with or without added grain concentrate free choice is an efficient, economic alternative to traditional hay/high NSC concentrate rations under the conditions of these trials. This type of ration may be especially appropriate for young horses that are predisposed to DOD. Anecdotal reports of use of TMR rations formulated for adult horses have been equally encouraging. With soaring prices for hay and, increasingly, grain in many regions of the world, the use of bagged TMR rations that can easily be transported and stored worldwide may be the most economic and practical answer for horse owners.

References

Flores RS, Byron CR, Kline KH (2009) Effects of feed type on average daily gain and gastric ulcer development in weanling horses. In: Proc Eq Sci Soc Symp, Keystone, CO, USA; Pp 152-155.

Frank N, Geor RJ, Bailey SR (2010) Equine metabolic syndrome. J Vet Internal Med 24:467-475.

National Research Council (1989) Nutrient requirements of horses. 5th edition. National Academy Press, Washington, DC, USA.

National Research Council (2007) Nutrient requirements of horses 6th ed National Academy Press, Washington, DC, USA.

Lewis LD (1995): Equine Clinical Nutrition. In: Feeding and Care. Williams and Wilkins, Philadelphia, USA; Chapter 15.

Pagan JD, Geor R, Caddel SE, Pryor PB, Hoekstra KE (2001) The Relationship Between Glycemic Response and the Incidence of OCD in Thoroughbred Weanlings: A Field Study. In: Proc Am Assoc Eq Pract 47; Pp 322-326.

Ralston SL (1996) Hyperglycemia/hyperinsulinemia after feeding a meal of grain to young horses with osteochondritis dissecans (OCD) lesions. Pferdeheilkunde 12:320-322.

Ralston SL (2002) Insulin and glucose regulation. Vet Clin North America Eq Pract: Endocrinology; Messer NT, Johnson PJ (eds) 18:295-304.

Ralston SL, Anderson H, Johnson R (2007a) Glucose/insulin responses of weanling horses fed forage based total mixed ration cubes versus hay/concentrate rations. In: Am Soc Anim Sci Joint Meeting, San Antonio, TX, USA, Abstract #61.

Ralston SL, Anderson H, Johnson R (2007b) Growth performance of draft cross weanlings fed forage based total mixed ration cubes versus traditional hay/grain rations. In: Proc Eq Sci Soc Symp, Hunt Valley, MD, USA; Pp 235-237.

Ralston SL, Anderson H, Johnson R (2007c) Growth and Glucose/insulin responses in draft cross weanlings fed Total Mixed Ration Cubes versus hay/concentrate rations. In. Applied Equine Nutrition and Training. Lindner A (ed), Wageningen Academic Publishers, Netherlands; Pp 233-239.

Ralston SL, Anderson H, Johnson R (2009) Growth response of draft cross weanlings fed 90% forage total mixed ration cubes versus traditional hay/concentrate rations. J Eq Vet Sci 29:386-387.

Treiber KH, Boston RC, Kronfeld DS, Staniar WB Harris PA (2005) Insulin resistance and compensation in Thoroughbred weanlings adapted to high-glycemic meals. J Anim Sci 83:2357-2364.

Valberg SJ, McCue ME, Mickelson JR (2011) The interplay of genetics, exercise and nutrition in polysaccharide storage myopathy. J Eq Vet Sci 31:205-210.

Warren SN, DePedro-Gonzalez P, Kline K (2011) Effects of feed form on growth and stomach ulcers. J Eq Vet Sci 31:330.

Williams CA, Urban C, Westendorf ML (2011) Dietary protein affects nitrogen and ammonia excretion in horses. J Eq Vet Sci 31:305-306.

Westendorf ML, Williams CA (2011) Effects of excess dietary phoshorus on fecal phosphorus excretion and water extractable phosphorus in horses. J Eq Vet Sci 31:306.

Expanded abstracts

Effect of a complementary horse feed on nervous horse behaviour

M. Barbier, S. Benoit and J.L. Lambey

Lambey, S.A., Moulin Des Prés, 71270 Torpes, France; barbier.martha@wanadoo.fr; s.benoit@lambey.fr

Take home message

Master CALM' horse feed reduced intensity of behavioural responses to startle and novelty reactions. Moreover, feeding horses with Master CALM' influenced heart rate parameters. The lower maximal heart rates and weaker increase percentages indicated a reduction of stress level. Horses were less excited and quickly calmed down after exposure to fearful situations.

Introduction

The environment of horses used for sport and leisure has changed from natural. Specific living conditions of the horse like stable containment involve movement restrictions and change their social relationships. Work subjection, transport, and competition go against the natural horse lifestyle. All these factors are stress sources for the horse and may have effects on his behaviour, induce uncontrolled reactions (shying, bolting...), and develop chronic stress in anxious horses (Forkman et al., 2007). Fear reactions seem to be more violent in nervous horses and cause physical injuries to himself and his user. These behavioural problems can also affect animal performance and spoil health (Hausberger et al., 2008, 2009). Previous studies have shown that diet could be a way to influence horse behaviour. The intake of large amounts of starch and sugars has been suggested to cause excitable behaviour (Redondo et al., 2009) whereas dietary fats could improve reactivity of horses (Holland et al., 1996) with comparable intake of digestible energy (McKenzie et al., 2003). In this context, we have developed a new complementary horse feed (Master CALM') which aims at calming nervous horses. The objective of this study was to assess the effect of Master CALM' on behaviour of nervous horses.

Materials and methods

Subjects and management

17 jumping horses from 11 French stables were selected for this study because they were considered as difficult to handle or to ride by stable manager, instructor, coach or their owner in comparison to others in the same stable. They were kept in 12 m^2 boxes. These horses performed as jumpers or event horses and maintained consistent work levels of 6-7 h/week throughout the study period.

Dietary treatment and experimental procedure

Horses were randomly allocated to 1 of the 2 diets that were tested in a parallel experimental design. They were fed with meadow hay complemented with concentrate in 2 or 3 meals depending on the stable (Table 1). The control diet consisted of the usual pelleted or flaked concentrate feed of the horses. The test diet consisted of Master CALM' (Lambey SA, Torpes, France). The 2 types of horse feed contained similar crude protein and carbohydrate contents, but differed in the fat and starch balance: control concentrate had on average 4.6% fat – 33.8% starch and Master CALM' 9.5% fat – 15% starch. Master CALM' horse feed is enriched with vitamins B1, B2, C, E, magnesium and tryptophan. The amount of Master CALM' was calculated to be iso-energetic to the usual concentrate they received before. Water was available ad libitum in the box. Horses were fed with their diet for 6 weeks before the behavioural tests were performed.

Tests of temperament

Our study focused on fear reactions which are defined as the horse capacity to react to the perception of potentially threatening reactions (Boissy, 1995; Forkman et al., 2007). Three behavioural tests were established to characterize fear reactions when horses were faced to novelty, suddenness or both. These tests were designed to measure fearfulness level of individuals and were always applied in the same order for all horses. The tests were standardized (sequence, duration, equipment, and operator) and they took place in the horse's box. Each test was performed only once in order to avoid habituation (Jones, 1988). The moment to perform the tests during the day was randomly

Table 1. Characteristics of animals and feeding practices in each group at the start of the study.

	Control group	Test group
Age	11±4 years (6 to 20 years)	9±3 years (8 to 15 years)
Sex	4 geldings, 5 mares	5 geldings, 3 mares
Weight	533±40 kg	498±41 kg
Breed	8 French Saddle horses	5 French Saddle horses
	1 Saddle horse	1 Anglo-arab
		1 Belgisch Warmbloed
		Paardenstamboek
		1 Saddle horse
Discipline	8 jumping horses	6 jumping horses
	1 eventing horses	2 school horses
Number of horsefeed meals per day	3 meals in 8 stables	3 meals in 5 stables
	2 meals in 1 stable	2 meals in 3 stables
Average of hay quantity (kg/day)	6.3±2.4	5±1.6
Average of horsefeed quantity (kg/day)	3.4±1.4	4±1.4
Bedding type	5 horses on straw	7 horses on straw
	3 horses on shavings	1 horse on sawdust
	1 horse on sawdust	

chosen for each horse in each group. Horses were quietly manipulated in their own boxes by the same person in each stable.

General procedures

Firstly, the horse's propensity to exhibit fear reactions when faced with novelty was tested using the tarpaulin test (Wolff *et al.* 1997; Nicol *et al.*, 2005). A bucket with food was put in a corner of a tarpaulin (1.90 × 1.60 m) spread out in a corner of the stall. Horse was compelled to walk on the tarpaulin in order to eat.

Then, the umbrella test was used to characterize horse's propensity to exhibit fear reactions when faced with suddenness (Holland *et al.*, 1996; Lansade, 2005). A colourful umbrella was abruptly opened 1 meter from horse's head.

Finally, the 'duck test' was used to characterize horse's propensity to exhibit fear reactions faced with novelty and suddenness (Wolff *et al.*, 1997). Concentrate food on a wooden tray was placed in a corner of the stall. The horse was left on its own in the stall for 3 min eating on the tray. Then, a plastic motorized duck was put on the tray. It began to turn and make noise for 20 s.

Behavioural observations

Behavioural observations were conducted using 2 observers with previous training of collecting behavioural data from horses. These observers were not blind to treatment. Horse behaviours were observed for 5 min and recorded on a cassette recorder by a cameraman for later analyses.

Horse posture reflects emotional status: eyes' expression and ears' position are signals used by the horse to express fear. Indeed, when a horse turns both ears forward and their eyes roll to the point that the white of the eye is visible, it indicates alertness (Trezzani, 2004). During the tarpaulin and the duck tests, vigilance posture occurrence for each horse was noted thanks to the observation of these 2 facial expressions.

Furthermore, the number of breaths was recorded during 5 min after stimulus. Breaths are emitted in case of danger (Trezzani, 2004) and are positively correlated with an alertness posture in horses (Lansade, 2005).

During the umbrella test, a reactivity score (Table 2) was assigned to the horse when opening the umbrella (Holland *et al.*, 1996). These scores allowed the evaluation of horse reactivity degree at the moment of the stimulus.

Physiological measurements

Fear-related reactions are characterized by physiological reactions preparing the animal to deal with the danger. When a stimulus occurs, an adrenaline release induces a heart rate increase. That is why heart rate was recorded by a heart rate monitor (Polar 625x, Polar Electro Europe BV, Fleurier, Switzerland) during the 3 tests (Mc Cann

Table 2. Score for observed reactions to a startling stimulus (Holland et al., 1996)

Score	Description
1	The horse shows no reaction or interest in the stimulus.
2	The horse looks in the direction of the stimulus but has no other reaction.
3	The horse jumps when the stimulus is applied but does not try to run away.
4	The horse jumps away from the stimulus and tries to leave.
5	The horse completely loses control and tries to flee or refuses to move from the spot.

et al., 1988a; Mc Cann *et al.*, 1988b; Harper, 1997; Strand *et al.*, 2002; Mckenzie *et al.*, 2003; Nicol *et al.*, 2005; Redondo *et al.*, 2009). Heart rate was recorded every 5 s from 3 min before to 5 min after stimulus. Data was processed with a Polar software package. Basal heart rate, maximum heart rate and time of return to basal heart rate have been recorded. Percentage of heart rate increase was calculated using basal heart rate and maximum heart rate data.

Statistical analysis

Regarding quantitative variables (heart rate, number of breaths), a comparison test of means between the 2 groups was chosen. It was made with Kruskal Wallis test, a nonparametric test (Excel, Microsoft). For qualitative data (alertness posture), a comparison between the 2 groups was performed using the Chi^2 Test with Excel software. The level of statistical significance was pre-set at $P < 0.05$.

Results

From a behavioural point of view

During the tarpaulin and duck tests, horses fed with the control diet gave out more breaths for 5 min than with the test diet (Table 3). During the tarpaulin test, 8/9 horses were in alert in the control group against only 1/8 in the test group (Table 3). For the duck test, no significant difference on alertness was observed among the horses consuming the different diets (Table 3).

Table 3. Effects of the diets on behavioural and physiological parameters of horses when faced with novelty or suddenness.

	Tarpaulin test			Umbrella test			Duck test		
	Control diet	Test diet	P values	Control diet	Test diet	P values	Control diet	Test diet	P values
Behavioural observations									
Number of breaths	9±9[a]	0±1[b]	0.0082				7±4[a]	3±4[b]	0.0153
Number of horses in alert	8[a]	1[b]	0.0016				9	6	NS
Reactivity score				4[a]	3[b]	0.0249			
Physiological measurements									
Maximum heart rate (beats/min)	64±19	44±5	NS	82±16[a]	57±17[b]	0.0160	78±15	67±15	NS
Time required to return to the basal heart rate (seconds)	184±109	146±38	NS	83±37[a]	46±16[b]	0.0095	ND[1]	ND	NS
Increase percentage of heart rate (beats/min)	53±32[a]	19±11[b]	0.0161	91±45[a]	35±26[b]	0.0124	73±25	59±37	NS

Values are means ± SE of 9 horses for control diet and 8 horses for Master CALM' diet.
[a,b] Means in rows with different superscripts are significantly different ($P < 0.05$).
[1] Not determined.

In response to the umbrella opening, horses appeared less reactive when consuming the test diet than consuming the control diet. Horses fed with the control diet jumped and tried to flee. They obtained on average a reactivity score of 4 out of 5 (Table 3). When fed with the test diet, horses only jumped without trying to escape and got on average a score of 3 which was significantly lower than for the control group (Table 3).

From a physiological point of view

In response to the umbrella, maximal heart rate was significantly lower in horses receiving the test diet than those receiving the control diet (Table 3). No significant difference was detected on maximum heart rate during the duck and tarpaulin tests.

A smaller percentage of heart rate increase was recorded in horses fed the test diet compared to those fed the control diet when they were excited by the tarpaulin and the umbrella (Table 3). Results were not significantly different between the 2 groups during the duck test. Finally, horses fed the test diet took a shorter time to return to their basal heart rate than horses fed the control diet during the umbrella test but no difference was observed during the tarpaulin test (Table 3).

Discussion and conclusion

The main difficulty encountered in this type of studies is the great variability among individuals as noticed by the standard deviations calculated. Indeed, besides diet composition, other factors like environment (type of housing, management...), genetic, sex and age could have had effects on the behaviour of the horses (Roche, 2008). The results confirm and extend those of earlier studies that investigated the influence of diet on horse behaviour. Diet composition can alter behavioural and physiological parameters related to stress and fearfulness reactions in horses (Holland *et al.*, 1996; McKenzie *et al.*, 2003; Redondo *et al.*, 2009).

In this study, the Master CALM' horse feed seems to have reduced intensity of behavioural responses to startle and novelty reactions. Horses showed weaker reactions when faced to novelty and suddenness and their alertness and reactivity levels were lower. Moreover, feeding horses with Master CALM' influenced heart rate parameters. The lower maximal heart rates and weaker increase percentages indicated a reduction of stress level. Horses were less excited and calmed down quicker after exposure to fearfulness situation.

Acknowledgement

This work is derived from an engineer thesis – Institut National Supérieur des Sciences Agronomiques de l'Alimentation et de l'Environnement (AGROSUP Dijon, France)

References

Boissy A (1995) Fear and fearfulness in determining behaviour. The Quarterly Review of Biology 70:165-191.

Forkman B, Boissy A, Meunier-Salaün MC, Canali E, Jones RB (2007) A critical review of fear tests used on cattle, pigs, sheep, poultry and horses. Physiology and Behavior 92:340-374.

Harper F (1997) Tryptophan for horses. J Eq Vet Sci 17: 357.

Hausberger M, Roche H, Henry S, Visser EK (2008) Synthèse sur la relation homme-cheval. Applied Animal Behaviour Science 109:1-24.

Hausberger M, Gautier E, Biquand V, Lunel C, Jégo P (2009) Could Work Be a Source of Behavioural Disorders? A Study in Horse. PLoS ONE 4:e7625.

Holland JL, Kronfeld DS, Meacham TN (1996) Behavior of horses is affected by soy lecithin and corn oil in the diet. J Anim Sci 74:1252-1255.

Jones RB (1988) Repeatability of fear ranks amoung adult laying hens. Appl Anim Behaviour Sci 19:297-304.

Lansade L (2005) Le tempérament du cheval. Etude théorique. Application à la sélection des chevaux destinés à l'équitation. Thèse de Doctorat Vétérinaire, Tours, Université de François Rabelais, 298 p.

Mc Cann JS, Heird JC, Bell RW, Lutherer LO (1988a) Normal and more highly reactive horses. I. Heart rate, respiration rate and behavioral observations. Appl Anim Behaviour 19:201-214.

Mc Cann JS, Heird JC, Bell RW, Lutherer LO (1988b) Normal and more highly reactive horses. II. The effects of handling and reserpine on the cardiac response to stimuli. Appl Anim Behaviour 19:215-226.

McKenzie EM, Valberg SJ, Godden SM, Pagan JD, MacLeay JM, Geor RJ, Carlson GP (2003) Effect of dietary starch, fat, and bicarbonate content on exercise responses and serum creatine kinase activity in equine recurrent exertional rhabdomyolysis. J Vet Internal Med 17:683-701.

Nicol CJ, Badnell-Waters AJ, Bice R, Kelland A, Wilson AD, Harris PA (2005) The effects of diet and weaning method on the behaviour of young horses. Appl Anim Behaviour Sci 95.205-221.

Redondo AJ, Carranza J, Trigo P (2009) Fat diet reduces stress and intensity of startle reaction in horses. Appl Anim Behaviour Sci 118:69-75.

Roche H (2008) Comportements et postures que devez-vous savoir observer. Belin, 125 p. (Connaissance du cheval) ISBN-2701141265.

Trezzani B (2004) Les phobies chez le cheval: élaboration d'un questionnaire d'enquête et présentation de cinq cas cliniques. Thèse de Doctorat Vétérinaire. Nantes, Université de Nantes, 210p.

Strand SC, Tiefenbacher S, Haskell M, Hosmer T, McDonnel SM, Freeman DA (2002) Appl Anim Behaviour Sci 78:145-157.

Wolff A (1997) Experimental tests to assess emotionality in horses. Behavioural Processes 40:209-221.

The effect of caecal pH on *in vivo* fibre digestibility in Norwegian trotter horses

C. Brøkner[1], D. Austbø[2], J.A. Næsset[2], K.E. Bach Knudsen[3] and A.H. Tauson[1,2]
[1]University of Copenhagen, Faculty of Life Sciences, Department of Basic Animal and Veterinary Sciences, Grønnegaardsvej 3, 1870 Frederiksberg C, Denmark; stinne@life.ku.dk
[2]Department of Animal and Aquacultural Sciences, Norwegian University of Life Sciences, Box 5003, 1432 Ås, Norway
[3]Aarhus University, Faculty of Science and Technology, Department of Animal Health and Bioscience, Research Centre Foulum, Blichers Allé 20, 830 Tjele, Denmark

Take home message

The take home message is that whole barley should be avoided in order not to lower caecal pH; although these results do not indicate an effect of low pH on fibre digestibility.

Introduction

Feeding 2 g barley starch per kg body weight (BW) in one meal has been shown to lower the caecal pH from around 7 to 6.1 (Austbø, 2005). Several studies have shown that replacing roughages with barley starch has resulted in decreased fibre digestibility (Julliand *et al.*, 2001, Drogoul *et al.*, 2001), supposedly due to decreased hindgut pH and switch in substrate from fibre to starch. This experiment aimed at quantifying the effect of caecal pH on fibre digestibility. It was hypothesised that decreased caecal pH would lower apparent fibre digestibility.

Material and methods

Experimental design

A Latin Square design with four dietary treatments, four periods and four horses was used to quantify the effect of caecal pH on fibre digestibility. Within each experimental period, a sequence of 17 days adaptation to the feed was followed by 2 consecutive sampling periods of each 4 days. The daily feed rations were divided into three meals and fed in the morning before sampling (at 6 am) and after end sampling in the afternoon (at 3.30 pm) and before the night (at 10 pm).

Animals

Four Norwegian Cold-blooded Trotter geldings (age 5-16 years) with an average BW of 544 kg and a mean body condition score of 6 on a scale from 1 to 9 were used. The horses were fitted with a permanent ceacal cannula close to the ileo-caecal junction. The horses were housed under the same conditions in individual 3 × 3 m stalls on wood shavings during the whole experimental period. The horses were exercised daily on a high-speed treadmill. The protocol consisted of a 10 min warm-up at 1.5-3.4 m/sec and 3% elevation followed by 8 min at 3.8 m/sec, 5 min at 4.2 m/sec and 3 min at 4.2 m/sec. A 1.5 min walk (1.8 m/sec) separated each sprint.

Diets

The daily amount of each feed type of the four experimental diets is seen in Table 1. The morning meal consisted of – in kg DM – 3.8 kg timothy hay (H), which served as control, 2.6 kg whole oats and 280 g sugar beet pulp coated with molasses (Betfor®) soaked in 1 L water + 1.6 kg timothy hay (OB), 1.9 kg whole barley and 280 g (dry weight) Betfor®, soaked in 1 L water + 1.6 kg timothy hay (BB), and 1.4 kg EquiGard® (a loose chaff based concentrate composed of: 24% hay, 22% apple pulp, 22% sugar beet pulp, 4.7% linseed; for more details http://en.hippolyt.com/Hauptfutter/Equigard.htm) + 1.6 kg timothy hay (M). The concentrate meals were fed at Time 1 and timothy hay 2 ½ h later. The remaining feed was divided into two meals and fed after sampling ended in the afternoon and before the night. The daily

Table 1. Daily amount of each feed type (kg DM) in the four diets.

Ingredients	Diets[1]			
	H[2]	OB[2]	BB[2]	M
Hay, kg DM	11.44	6.45	6.45	6.45
Oats, kg DM	-	2.58	-	-
Barley, kg DM	-	-	2.04	-
Betfor, kg DM	-	0.85	0.85	-
Equigard®, kg DM	-	-	-	4.24
DM intake, kg	11.44	9.88	9.34	10.68

[1] H (Hay), OB (Oats and Betfor®), BB (barley and Betfor®) and M (EquiGard®).
[2] The diets were fortified with a mineral and vitamin supplement.

ration fulfilled Danish feeding standards for horses at medium (1.5 × maintenance) work level.

Sampling

A pH electrode, attached to a logger, was inserted to the caecum through the cannula and pH was recorded at 1 min intervals for 9 hours starting before the morning meal at 6:00 h. The horses were fitted with a harness for total collection of faeces. Faeces were collected for 4 days, pooled and mixed thoroughly before a representative sample was stored at -20 °C before analysis. Feeds were analysed for neutral detergent fibre (NDF), non-starch polysaccharides (NSP), soluble non-cellulosic polysaccharides (S-NCP) and insoluble non-cellulosic polysaccharides (I-NCP) and faeces were analysed for NSP, S-NCP and I-NCP as described by Brøkner *et al.* (2010a).

Statistical analyses

The pH recordings from each measurements series (horse*diet) were averaged over 1 hour intervals. A polynomial shape for the pH profiles was evaluated by analysis of variance using the MIXED procedure in SAS version 9.2 with horse as random effect. The final model used was:

$Y_{ijk} = \mu + \alpha(\text{diet}_i) + \beta(\text{diet}_i * \text{time}_j) + \gamma(\text{diet}_i * \text{time}_j^2) + \delta(\text{horse}_k) + \varepsilon(\text{residual error}_{ijk})$

where $i = 1 - 4$; $j = 1 - 9$; $k = 1 - 4$. The fibre digestibility was statistically evaluated by analysis of variance using the PROC GLM procedure in SAS version 9.2 with feed and period as fixed effects and horse as random effect in the model. The model used was:

$y_{ij}(\text{digestibility}) = \mu + \alpha(\text{feed}_i) + \beta(\text{period}_j) + \varepsilon(\text{residuals})_{ij}$

where; $i = 1 - 4$; $j = 1 - 4$. A *P*-value less than 0.05 was considered significant.

Results and discussion

The lowest pH was 6.62 for H, 6.56 for OB, 6.47 for BB and 6.64 for M and was recorded 5 hours postprandially after which, caecal pH began to rise (Figure 1). Whole barley fed in combination with Betfor® lowered the caecal pH significantly ($P < 0.001$) more than H, OB and M diets (Figure 1). The OB diet lowered the caecal pH more as compared to H and M diets; however, the three diets did not differ significantly. There was an overall dietary effect ($P < 0.001$) on lowering caecal pH; however, there was no correlation between low pH and fibre digestibility. One explanation is that the caecal pH did not remain low long enough to influence fibre digestibility. Furthermore, the fall in pH did not reach the expected low level of 6.1 as previously reported by Austbø (2005) after feeding barley to horses. A likely reason is, as discussed by Brøkner *et al.* (2010b), that beet pulp fed in combination with whole unprocessed barley prevented a fall in caecal pH. The effect of more feed ingredients in preventing a fall in caecal pH is supported by the results of the M diet, where caecal pH remained around 6.65 throughout the whole sampling period.

There was a strong dietary effect ($P < 0.01$) on apparent digestibility (AD) of S-NCP, which ranged from 82 to 86% in BB, OB and M compared to 41% in H (Table 2). The difference is most likely explained by the high content of easily accessible uronic acid in beet and apple pulps. In general the AD of organic matter (OM), S-NCP and cellulose was lowest for the H diet, which can be explained by the lower content of soluble fibre and high lignin content in hay (Brøkner *et al.*, 2010a). AD

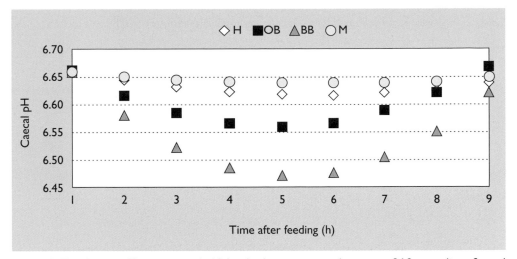

Figure 1. The dietary effect on caecal pH (each plot represents the mean of 60 recordings from 4 horses). The concentrate meals were fed at Time 1 and hay at Time 2.5. H (Hay), OB (Oats and Betfor®), BB (Barley and Betfor®) and M (EquiGard®).

of cellulose ranged between 55 to 59%. Cellulose is primarily associated with forages, which explains the lack of dietary effect ($P=0.32$), as all horses were fed the same type of hay. The NDF digestibility was significantly ($P=0.05$) affected by diet and was highest for M and H (56%) as compared to OB (52%) and BB (54%). This is supposedly explained by the higher content of indigestible arabinoxylans in the aleuron and husk layers of the two cereals (Bach Knudsen, 2001). The AD of NSP ranged from 55% in H up to 62% in M; however, diets only tended to affect fibre digestibility. NSP includes the indigestible NCP fraction and the lack of dietary effect is most likely explained by the lignin content in hay and indigestible fibre fractions in cereals. The digestibility of I-NCP was lowest for OB and BB (5%) but did not differ significantly between diets ($P=0.34$). As expected, OM had the highest digestibility (ranged between 60 and 65%) as this part besides carbohydrates also includes fat and protein. As expected the NDF fraction was less digestible than NSP, which supposedly is caused by the method of analysis; lignin is included in the NDF analysis and not in the NSP analysis (Table 2). Additionally, most S-NCP is lost in the NDF procedure.

C. Brøkner, D. Austbø, J.A. Næsset, K.E. Bach Knudsen and A.H. Tauson

Table 2. The apparent fibre digestibility as a percentage of dry matter of different diets.

	Diets[2]				
	H	OB	BB	M	P-value
OM[1]	60[a]	65[b]	65[b]	65[b]	0.02
NSP[1]	55[a]	56[a]	56[a]	62[b]	0.10
S-NCP[1]	41[a]	85[b]	82[b]	86[b]	<0.01
I-NCP[1]	8	5	5	11	0.34
Cellulose	55	55	55	59	0.32
NDF[1]	56[a]	52[b]	54[ba]	56[a]	0.05

[1] Organic matter (OM), Non-starch polysaccharide (NSP), soluble non-cellulosic polysaccharides (S-NCP), insoluble non-cellulosic polysaccharides (I-NCP) and neutral detergent fibre (NDF).
[2] H (Hay), OB (Oats and Betfor®), BB (Barley and Betfor®) and M (EquiGard®).

Conclusion

The lowest caecal pH was recorded 5 hours postprandial and was significantly lowest in the Barley/Betfor® diet compared to the three other experimental diets. Unexpectedly, the apparent fibre digestibility was unaffected by the low caecal pH. The take home message is that whole barley should be avoided in order not to lower caecal pH; although these results do not indicate an effect of low pH on fibre digestibility.

Acknowledgement

The authors would like to acknowledge Nordic Sugar A/S, St. Hippolyt Denmark A/S and the Danish Directorate for Development for financial support.

References

Austbø D (2005) pH-verdien i blindtarmen hos hest, effekt av rasjon og tid. Husdyrforsøksmøtet, Norway.

Bach Knudsen KE (2001) The nutritional significance of 'dietary fibre' analysis. Anim Feed Sci Technol 90:3-20.

Brøkner C, Bach Knudsen KE, Tauson AH (2010) Fibre content and physiochemical properties of various horse feed ingredients. Proc of the 1st Nordic Feed Science Conference, Uppsala, Sweden. Pp 107–111.

Brøkner C, Austbø D, Næsset JA, Bach Knudsen KE, Tauson AH (2010b) The effect of sugar beet pulp on caecal pH in Norwegian cold-blooded trotter horses. In: The impact of nutrition on the health and welfare of horses. Ellis AD, Longland AC, Coenen M, Miraglia N (eds). Wageningen Academic Publishers, Wageningen, The Netherlands. Pp 210-212.

Drogoul C, de Fombelle A, Julliand V (2001) Feeding and microbial disorders in horses: 2: Effect of three hay:grain ratios on digesta passage rate and digestibility in ponies. J Eq Vet Sci 21:487-491.

Julliand V, de Fombelle A, Drogoul C, Jacotot E (2001) Feeding and microbial disorsers in horses: part 3 – effects of three hay:grain ratios on microbial profile and activities. J Eq Vet Sci 21:543-546.

Effect of 5 week training period on the glycemic and insulinemic response to a cereal meal in Standardbreds

A.G. Goachet[1], C. Philippeau[1], V.J. Adams[2], V. Julliand[1] and P. Harris[3]
[1]URANIE, 26 bd Dr Petitjean, BP 87999, 21079 Dijon Cedex, France; ag.goachet@agrosupdijon.fr
[2]Veterinary Epidemiology Consultant, Suffolk, United Kingdom
[3]Equine Studies Group – WALTHAM Center for Pet Nutrition, Melton Mowbury, Leics, LE14 4RT, United Kingdom

Take home message

In healthy Standardbreds, a 5 week period of training is associated with a decreased glucose response to an oat challenge test, even after 6 days of inactivity. This suggests a more permanent increase in insulin sensitivity.

Introduction

In man, physical activity has a beneficial effect on insulin sensitivity (IS) (Henriksson, 1995). There is, however, a distinction between the acute effects of exercise and genuine training effects (Borghouts and Keizer, 2000). Up to two hours after exercise, glucose uptake is in part elevated due to insulin independent mechanisms and a single bout of exercise can increase insulin sensitivity for at least 16 hours post-exercise. Physical training potentiates the effect of exercise on insulin sensitivity through multiple adaptations in glucose transport and metabolism (Borghouts and Keizer, 2000).

In horses, some recent studies have examined the relationship between physical activity and IS (Pratt et al., 2006; De Graaf-Roelfsema et al., 2006; Stewart-Hunt et al., 2006; 2010). Whilst there may be evidence that exercise leads to an increase in IS, the results concerning the effects of a long-term training period appear to be variable. Two studies for example (Pratt et al., 2006; De Graaf-Roelfsema et al., 2006) concluded that 7 and 18 weeks of training respectively did not result in a change in glucose metabolism or IS when evaluated 3 days after the last bout of exercise. However, Stewart-Hunt *et al.* (2010) observed an improvement of IS after 7 week physical training in Standardbreds, which persisted after 3 days of inactivity.

The aim of this study was to determine the effects of a 5 week training period, and a subsequent period of inactivity (6 days) on the glycemic and insulinemic response in previously inactive Standardbred horses. Because our horses were in a training center, we selected a technique to evaluate the glucose and insulin response which is comparatively easy to undertake in practice: the oral Oat Challenge Test (OCT) (as compared with the euglycaemic-hyperinsulinemic clamp or the frequently sampled intravenous glucose tolerance test).

Material and methods

Eight untrained Standardbred geldings aged 4.9 ± 1.5 years, with a body weight (BW) of 496 ± 32 kg, and a body condition score (BCS) of 3.3 ± 0.2 (on a scale of 0 to 5 according to the method of INRA-HN-IE, 1997) were used. All horses had not undergone forced exercise for one year prior to the study, having being maintained out in paddocks over this time period. During the study, horses were housed in 4 × 3.5 m free stalls, on artificial bedding. They were put into paddocks for several hours a day for free exercise. They were fed hay and a pelleted concentrate (SPILLERS performance cubes) (Table 1). Hay was provided in 2 equal meals at 10:00 and 16:00 h, concentrate in 3 equal meals, at 8:00, 12:00 and 17:30 h. Salt blocks and water were available *ad libitum*. For 7 days before the evaluations were carried out, horses were fed exactly 2.1% BW DM in a ratio of 54:46 (H:C). For the remainder of the study, they were fed at 2-2.3% BW DM in a ratio of 55:45 (H:C). Horses were weighed and their BCS recorded weekly throughout the study.

After 3 weeks of dietary adaptation and before the start of training (P1), an oat challenge test (OCT1) was undertaken in all horses. Then, 6 horses were chosen by the trainer to go into training (T) and the other 2 remained as non-exercising controls (C). The 2 C horses (4 years old; 485 and 526 kg; BCS 3.3 and 3) remained in the paddock. The T horses (5.2 ± 1.6 years old; 492 ± 35 kg; BCS 3.3 ± 0.4) were driven 2 times a week on a 1150 m sandy track, according to a training program

Table 1. Biochemical composition of the feeds.

	Hay	Pelleted feed
OM (%DM)	91.9	92.7
NDF (%DM)	64.0	26.8
ADF (%DM)	34.8	11.5
ADL (%DM)	4.6	2.6
Cellulose (%DM)	30.2	8.9
Hemicellulose (%DM)	29.1	15.3
CP (%DM)	7.0	15.4
Starch (% DM)	<1.0	26.8
Fat (% DM)	<1.0	5.4
GE (kcal/g DM)	4.01	4.48

consisting of both continuous exercise (CE) and interval running (IT), which increased in intensity over the 5 week study period (Table 2). After 5 weeks, the OCT (OCT2) was then repeated on all 8 horses. OCT2 was performed after a 6 days period of inactivity (stall resting only).

OCTs were performed with four horses being evaluated each day. Feed was withheld 12 hours prior to the beginning of the test. A series of blood samples was then collected via a venous jugular catheter at -30, -5, 10, 30, 50, 60, 90, 120, 150, 180, 210, 240, 300 and 360 min after a 1.5 kg as fed meal of rolled oats (87.2% DM; 28.2% starch – same batch used for each evaluation) given at time 0. Blood samples were collected

Table 2. Training program for the Trained group.

Week 1	Exercise 1	3 km CE @ 5.5 m/sec
	Exercise 2	3 km CE @ 5.5 m/sec
Week 2	Exercise 1	3 km CE @ 5.5 m/sec
	Exercise 2	6 km CE @ 5.5 m/sec
Week 3	Exercise 1	6 km CE @ 5.5 m/sec
	Exercise 2	IT 4 km at 20 km/h plus 1 km at 9.7 m/sec
Week 4	Exercise 1	6 km CE @ 5.5 m/sec
	Exercise 2	IT 3 km at 20 km/h plus 2 km at 9.7 m/sec
Week 5	Exercise 1	6 km CE @ 5.5 m/sec
	Exercise 2	IT 2 km at 20 km/h plus 3 km at 9.7 m/sec

into fluoride oxalate tubes for glucose analysis and plain tubes for insulin. Intake time was recorded and any residual oats were removed after 30 min. Blood samples were immediately centrifuged at $1,600 \times g$ for 10 min, and plasma (glucose) or serum (insulin) was removed and stored at -20 °C until analysis. Plasma glucose concentrations were determined by the glucose oxidase method using a RX Imola chemical autoanalyzer (kit GLUC-PAP). Serum insulin was determined by a solid phase, enzyme-labeled chemiluminescent assay (Immulite Insulin Assay).

The magnitude of each glucose and insulin response was calculated as the incremental area under the curve (AUC_{GLU} and AUC_{INS}, respectively) by graphical approximation from summed trapezoids. Mean ± SD values for oats intake, glucose and insulin baseline concentration, peak concentration, time to peak concentration and AUC were calculated for the trained horses as well as for the 2 additional control horses. A linear mixed model was used to evaluate the effect of group (T vs C) on the glucose and insulin responses from the OCTs using the equation P2 = P1 + Group + sampling time to control for repeated measures. Using the trained horses as their own control, this analysis was repeated using the equation P2 = P1 + sampling time.

Results and conclusions

Horses BW and BCS remained constant throughout the study. At OCT1, 5 of the 8 horses did not eat the entire oat meal within the 30 min allocated time. For these horses, the amount of oats offered was then adjusted for OCT2, to be the same as consumed at OCT1. However, one of the trained horses (horse B) did not consume all the amended oat meal at OCT2 and the data were therefore evaluated with and without his results. For the T group, oats intake was 1.1 ± 0.4 kg as fed for OCT1 and OCT2, respectively. For Control Horse 1, oats intake was 1.5 kg as fed for OCT1 and OCT2. For Control Horse 2, oats intake was 1.0 and 0.6 kg as fed at OCT1 and OCT2 respectively. The average starch intake was 0.5-0.6 g DM/kg BW.

Basal glucose and insulin concentrations were within the normal physiological range (Table 3). The glucose and insulin responses (peak concentrations, AUC and time to peak) were in accordance with reported data obtained for a similar starch intake (Vervuert et al., 2009).

Table 3. Mean ± SD baseline concentrations of glucose and insulin, area under the glucose (AUC$_{GLU}$) and insulin (AUC$_{INS}$) curve values, peak glucose and insulin concentrations, and time to peak before (OCT1) and after 5-weeks (OCT2) of training and individual values for the 2 additional control horses (Control 1 and Control 2) which did not perform the training program.

	Trained group (n=6)		Control 1		Control 2	
	OCT 1	OCT 2	OCT1	OCT2	OCT1	OCT2
Baseline glucose (mmol/l)	4.9±0.1	5.0±0.3	4.6	4.4	4.9	5.2
Peak glucose (mmol/l)	8.5±0.5[a]	6.9±0.7[b]	7.3	7.4	5.4	5.4
Time to peak glucose (min)	105±25	95±29	150	90	150	120
AUC$_{GLU}$ (mmol/l/min)	527±152[a]	189±107[b]	500	461	46	29
Baseline insulin (µIU/ml)	2.1±1.9	2.9±2.6	0.5	0.5	0.5	2.9
Peak insulin (µIU/ml)	92.7±84.0	45.5±24.8	100	140	3.4	5.2
Time to peak insuline (min)	170±45[a]	110±24[b]	180	180	120	180
AUC$_{INS}$ (µIU/ml/min)	13,457±14,026	5,793±3,239	13,911	17,894	491	177

[a,b] Means in rows with different superscripts are significantly different ($P<0.05$).

A training effect was observed on the glycemic response (Figure 1) but not on the insulin response, as shown by the significantly lower AUC$_{GLU}$ and peak glucose observed after 5 weeks of training in the T group but not in the C group (Table 3). The same results were seen whether horse B was included or excluded in the analysis. The effect on the glucose response was observed after a 6 day period of inactivity, which is in accordance with previous data obtained following 3 and 5 days of inactivity in trained Standardbreds (Stewart-Hunt *et al.*, 2006; 2010). This suggests an effect of physical training on IS. However, this decreased glucose response in comparison to normal could be related to alterations in other parameters such as individual starch digestion and glucose absorption. Large individual variations were observed for

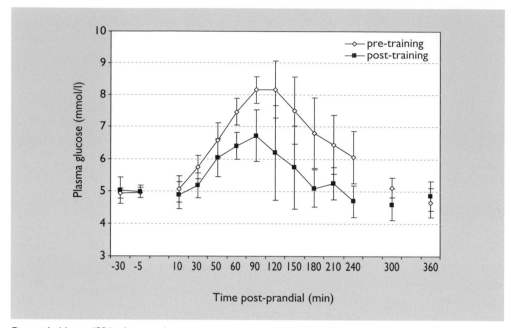

Figure 1. Mean (SD) plasma glucose concentrations (mmol/l) before and after 5-weeks of training in Standarbreds.

AUC_{GLU}, AUC_{INS} and insulin peak. This has already been reported by Hoffman *et al.* (2003) who calculated 88% individual variation in the glycemic response after an OCT. Nevertheless, the variation in glycemic and insulinemic response to a particular feed may be more related to individual variation in systemic regulation of glucose and insulin, than to individual variation in digestion and absorption (Staniar *et al.*, 2009). This needs further investigation.

Acknowledgements

This study was supported by the WALTHAM Centre for Pet Nutrition and AgroSup Dijon. Authors acknowledge all the people of AgroSup for the care of the horses and the laboratory analysis; Sébastien and Thierry Collaud for the training of horses; Robert Cash, from Beaufort Cottage Laboratory, for his advice about insulin data.

References

Borghouts LB, Keizer HA (2000) Exercise and insulin sensitivity: a review. Int J Sports Med 21:1-12.

De Graaf-Roelfsema E, Ginneken ME, Breda E, Wijnberg ID, Keizer HA, van der Kolk JH (2006) The effect of long-term exercise on glucose metabolism and peripheral insulin sensitivity in Standarbred horses. Equine vet J Suppl 36:221-225.

Henriksson J (1995) Influence of exercise on insulin sensitivity. Journal of Cardiovascular Risk 2:303-309.

Hoffman RM (2003) Carbohydrate metabolism in horses. In: Recent advances in equine nutrition. Ralston SL, Hintz HF (Eds). International Veterinary Information Service, Ithaca, New-York, USA.

INRA-HN-IE (1997) Notation de l'état corporel des chevaux de selle et de sport. Guide pratique. Institut de l'élevage, Paris, France.

Pratt SE, Geor RJ, McCutcheon LJ (2006) Effects of dietary energy source and physical conditioning on insulin sensitivity and glucose tolerance in Standardbred horses. Equine vet J Suppl 36:579-584.

Staniar WB, Grube HS, Jedrzejewski EA (2009) Inter-animal variation in glycemic and insulinemic responses to different carbohydrates sources. J Eq Vet Sci 29:377-379.

Stewart-Hunt L, Geor RJ, McCutcheon LJ (2006) Effects of short-term training on insulin sensitivity and skeletal muscle glucose metabolism in Standarbred horses. Equine vet J Suppl 36:226-232.

Stewart-Hunt L, Pratt-Philips S, McCutcheon LJ, Geor RJ (2010) Dietary energy source and physical conditioning affect insulin sensitivity and skeletal muscle glucose metabolism in horses. Equine vet J Suppl 42:355-360.

Vervuert I, Voigt K, Hollands T, Cuddeford D, Coenen M (2009) Effect of feeding increasing quantities of starch on glycaemic and insulinaemic responses in healthy horses. Vet J 182:67-72.

The use of equine K4b^2 during incremental field exercise tests in driven Standardbred trotters: a preliminary study

A.G. Goachet[1], J. Fortier[1,2], V. Julliand[1], H. Assadi[2] and R. Lepers[2]
[1]URANIE, 26 bd Dr Petitjean, BP 87999, 21079 Dijon Cedex, France; ag.goachet@agrosupdijon.fr
[2]Faculté des Sciences du Sport, Université de Bourgogne, BP 27877, 21078 Dijon, France

Take home message

The equine K4b^2 system is well tolerated by horses and allows O_2 and CO_2 measurements in field conditions up to maximal workload. The relationship between maximal oxygen consumption (VO_{2max}) and maximal aerobic speed (MAS) still needs to be established.

Introduction

As in human athletes (Levine, 2005), measurement of oxygen consumption (VO_2) in field conditions might be an appropriate way to approach energy expenditure (EE) in horses. Measurement of VO_2 during exercise is an accurate indicator of exercise intensity and could help to categorize the requirements of horses competing in different disciplines. In addition, VO_{2max}, i.e. the upper limit of the oxygen uptake, corresponds to the maximal aerobic capacity of the horses. To date, VO_2 and VO_{2max} measurements in exercising horses have been mostly done during treadmill tests (Evans, 2007) due to the lack of validated portable devices.

The equine K4b^2 is a portable system which allows continuous measurements of VO_2, CO_2 production (VCO_2), and heart rate (HR) in field conditions. This device has been tested successfully in saddle horses (Votion et al., 2006) and endurance horses (Cottin et al., 2010), but has shown some limits when used in driven Standardbred trotters (van Erck *et al.*, 2007). The first limitation is associated with the difficulty of driving horses with a hackamore, particularly at high speeds. The facemask has indeed been adapted to a hackamore bridle to allow control of the horse whilst ensuring air tightness. The second limitation is related to the difficulty of reaching VO_{2max} during field exercise tests. van Erck *et al.* (2007) suggested that the type of incremental exercise test applied in their study was inadequate to reach VO_{2max}. Indeed, the horses were allowed to recover at a slow trot for 2 min between each step. The authors also questioned the capacity of the system to measure accurately VO_2 at maximal levels of exercise. A continuous incremental exercise test might be a solution and the determination of the MAS (Maximal Aerobic Speed) could be an alternative parameter to predict VO_{2max}. The MAS is the velocity corresponding to the achievement of VO_{2max}. Commonly used in human activities (Billat and Koralsztein, 1996), MAS could quantify the exercise load during a training period, for example by expressing running speed as a percentage of the MAS.

The aims of this preliminary study were: (1) to assess the feasibility of VO_2 measurements using the equine $K4b^2$ and Equimask in driven Standardbred trotters in field conditions; (2) to evaluate a new exercise test protocol to reach VO_{2max} and MAS.

Material and methods

Six driven Standarbred geldings (from 4 to 7 years old, 495 ± 47 kg) underwent a regular trotting training program based on interspersing long and short intermittent workouts on an 1,150 m sandy track.

After three weeks of adaptation to the Equimask, horses were submitted to a track exercise test (TET). The TET was a continuous incremental exercise test consisting in consecutive 3 minutes steps at increasing speeds, up to exhaustion: the initial velocity was 4.2 m/s, and the increment was 1.4 m/s between steps. The speed was controlled by the driver with a GPS logger (Geonaute Keymaze 300). The TET was performed with the horses harnessed to a sulky, equipped by the $K4b^2$ system (Cosmed) and HR Polar (Equine Polar RS 800 CX G3). The hackamore bridle was replaced by a bit. Before each test, the O_2 and CO_2 analyzers were calibrated and a pre-test was done to establish a delay calibration between airflow and gas signals. During each TET, velocity (v), HR, VO$_2$ and VCO$_2$ were recorded. A blood sample was taken from the jugular vein before and within 3 minutes after the end of the last step for blood lactate concentration determination.

The captured data were downloaded to a PC using the K4b^2 management data software. VO$_2$, VCO$_2$ and HR data were filtered and averaged on 5 seconds, and transferred on Excel files to calculate RER (Respiratory Exchange Ratio) and VCO$_2$ (l/min)/VO$_2$ (l/min). Results of the breath-by-breath data were averaged over the 30 s during a steady-state period at the end of each step. Mean $\pm$ SD were calculated for each variable (VO$_2$, VCO$_2$, HR and RER) at each step.

Results and conclusions

All horses tolerated well the Equimask and completed the TET. The use of a bit instead of a hackamore bridle allowed a good control of the horses speed without interfering with the mask airtightness. To improve the security of the system, the K4b^2 analyzer was fixed on the sulky instead of to a strap fastened around the horse's thorax, as done by van Erk et al. (2007). Nevertheless, we faced another technical problem related to excessive head movements of horses. In particular, one horse knocked the Equimask on the ground which, by damaging the turbines, probably explains the incomplete VO$_2$ and VCO$_2$ recordings obtained for four horses. The use of a headcheck seems to be essential to limit excessive head movements and to ensure a maximal security of the Equimask.

HR and VO$_2$ values recorded at each step were consistent with previous data obtained from field exercise tests in Saddle horses (Hanak et al., 2001; Votion et al., 2006) and endurance horses (Cottin et al., 2010) using portable devices (Table 1). The VCO$_2$ values observed in our study were not markedly underestimated, contrary to those reported by Votion et al. (2006) and van Erck et al. (2007). As a consequence, we found RER greater than 1 (Table 1), whereas the calculated RER was inferior to 1 at all levels of exercise in previous studies.

HR$_{peak}$ values were close to those obtained by van Erck et al. (2007) (Table 2). A plateau of HR was observed during the last step for all horses, suggesting that HR$_{max}$ was reached. Except for horse 2, the blood lactate concentrations were particularly higher than those

Table 1. Physiological variables measured during the incremental exercise test according to the speed (mean ± SD; n=number of horses).

	Running speed at trot (m/s)					
	4.2	5.5	7.0	8.3	9.7	11.1
HR (bpm)	121±8 (n=6)	138±5 (n=6)	160±7 (n=6)	187±14 (n=6)	203±8 (n=5)	213±8 (n=4)
VO_2 (ml/min/kg)	43.6±7.2 (n=5)	51.8±1.3 (n=4)	62.0±8.9 (n=4)	75.8±7.8 (n=4)	105 (n=1)	128 (n=1)
VCO_2 (ml/min/kg)	35.5±6.9 (n=5)	41.5±1.2 (n=4)	53.3±8.7 (n=4)	67.1±9.0 (n=4)	101 (n=1)	129 (n=1)
RER	0.81±0.03 (n=5)	0.8±0.03 (n=4)	0.86±0.03 (n=4)	0.88±0.05 (n=4)	0.97 (n=1)	1.01 (n=1)

HR, heart rate; VO_2, volume of oxygen consumed; VCO_2, volume of carbon dioxide released; RER, calculated respiratory gas exchange ratio.

Table 2. Individual physiological variables measured at the end of the incremental exercise test.

Horse	Age years	Last step velocity m/sec	HR_{peak} bpm	La mmol/l	VO_{2peak} ml/min/kg	VCO_{2peak} ml/min/kg
1	5	11.1	223	21.8	132	135
2	4	8.3	223	6.0	85	85
3	7	11.1	226	23.7	-	-
4	6	11.1	213	15.9	-	-
5	7	11.1	221	16.8	-	-
6	5	11.1	224	23.7	-	-

Last step velocity, velocity at the last step completed; HR_{peak}, maximal HR recorded during the exercise test; La, blood lactate concentration at the end of the exercise test; VO_{2peak}, maximal value for oxygen consumption recorded during the exercise test; VCO_{2peak}, maximal value of carbon dioxide production recorded during the exercise test.

described by van Erck *et al.* (2007): 20.4 ± 3.7 *vs* 7.3 ± 3.0 respectively. The velocity reached at the last completed step was 8.3 m/s for Horse 2 and 11.1 for all other horses, which is consistent with van Erck *et al.* (2007). Regarding the VO_2 values of horse 1, a steady state was achieved at the end of the TET, indicating that this particular horse had reached VO_{2max} (Figure 1). The HR plateaus, the high concentrations of blood lactate and the fact that horses could not maintain higher speed suggest that the TET allowed them to reach maximal workload and probably MAS. However, due to the lack of VO_2 and VCO_2 data we cannot draw conclusions on VO_{2max}.

Further investigations are needed to confirm the relationship between MAS and VO_{2max} i.e to verify that when the horses reach their MAS, they also reach their VO_{2max}. In the future, those measurements could allow quantifying the EE of driven Standardbred horses during races and training, particularly the relative contribution of the aerobic and anaerobic systems. The accurate quantification of EE could help to better take into account the energetic nutritional requirements of driven Standardbred horses.

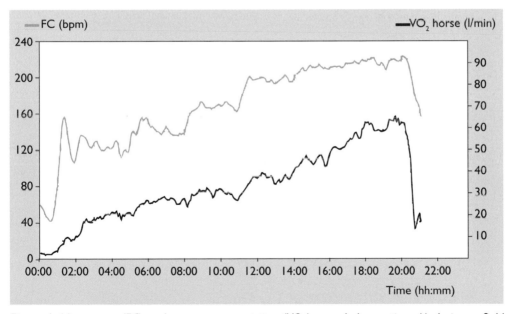

Figure 1. Heart rate (FC) and oxygen consumption (VO_2) recorded over time (t) during a field incremental exercise test of a representative horse (Horse 1).

Acknowledgements

This study was supported by INRA PHASE and AgroSup Dijon. Authors acknowledge the animal keepers at AgroSup for the care of the horses. They are also very grateful to Sébastien and Thierry Collaud for the horses training.

References

Billat V, Koralsztein JP (1996) Significance of the velocity at VO_{2max} and time to exhaustion at this velocity. Sports Med 22:90-108.

Cottin F, Metayer N, Goachet AG, Julliand V, Slawinski J, Billat V, Barrey E (2010) Oxygen consumption and gait variables of Arabian endurance horses measured during a field exercise test. Equine vet J Suppl 38:1-5.

Evans (2007) Physiology of equine performance and associated tests of function. Equine vet J 39:373-383.

Hanak J, Jahn P, Kabes R, Sedlinska M, Zert Z, Mezerova J, Chvatal O (2001) A field study of oxygen consumption and estimated energy expenditure in the exercising horse. Acta Vet Brno 70:133-139.

Levine JA (2005) Measurement of energy expenditure. Public Health Nutrition 8:1123-1132.

Van Erck E, Votion DM, Serteyn D, Art T (2007) Evaluation of oxygen consumption during field exercise tests in Standarbred trotters. Eq Comp Exerc Physiol 4:43-49.

Votion DM, Caudron I, Lejeune JP, Van der Heyden L, Art T, van Erck E, Serteyn D (2006) New perspectives for field measurement of cardiorespiratory parameters in exercising horses. Pferdeheilkunde 5: 619-624.

Applied equine nutrition and training

The effects of a high starch, cereal-based diet compared to a low starch, fibre-based diet on reactivity in horses

C.E. Hale[1], A.J. Hemmings[2] and S.E. Bee[1]
[1]Allen & Page Ltd, Norfolk Mill, Shipdham, Thetford, Norfolk, IP25 7SD, United Kingdom; chale@allenandpage.co.uk
[2]The Royal Agricultural College, Stroud Road, Cirencester, Gloucestershire, GL7 6JS, United Kingdom

Take home message

Horses fed on concentrate feeds which contain low starch (7%), show reduced reactivity compared to horses fed an isocalorific diet containing high levels of starch (28%).

Introduction

Horses have evolved as herd-dwelling, free-ranging, trickle feeders, which are physiologically designed to consume high fibre, low starch diets. Through modern management practices, brought about as a consequence of domestication, many modern-day equids develop abhorrent behaviours that may be linked to inappropriate management regimes. It has been suggested that traditional feeding practices centred around the provision of relatively low fibre, high starch diets may be implicated in the development of such undesirable behaviours (Hothersall and Nicol, 2009). Diets high in starch have been shown to elicit an increased glycaemic response (Williams et al., 2001), and indeed may, in turn, influence behaviour and reactivity (Ralston, 2007; Zeyner et al., 2004; Holland et al., 1996). The aim of this study is to consider the reactivity of horses fed either a high fibre, low starch concentrate diet, compared to a high starch, low fibre concentrate diet.

Materials and methods

Eight (n = 8) mature horses of varying breeds were used in the current study. The treatment animals consisted of five geldings and 3 mares and ranged in age between 6 and 14 years (average age 9.6 yrs). All horses were assessed to have a moderate body condition score and weights ranged from 287 kg to 805 kg (mean 441 kg). All horses were in light work and were kept on the same yard, housed in standard 3.65 × 3.65 m stables. Each horse was ridden for 40 minutes 5 times per week, achieving an average heart rate of 82 bpm. In addition to their ridden work, each horse was turned out in dirt paddocks for five hours each day.

Horses were randomly assigned to two treatment groups: treatment S (high starch feed; source was barley, maize and peas) or treatment F (high fibre feed; source was sugar beet, grass, straw, oat fibre). Both treatment diets were isocalorific and contained 9 MJ DE/kg. Treatment S contained 28% starch and 14% fibre and treatment F contained 7% starch and 24% fibre. All horses were fed according to weight and workload, as recommended by NRC (2007). Each horse received the concentrate portion of their ration in two meals at 7 am and 5 pm, with hay fed at 7 am, 3 pm and 5 pm.

Horses were fed each diet for a total of four weeks. At the end of the first treatment period, each group was transferred to the second treatment diet over a one week cross-over period. Basal heart rate was recorded during one hour/day over 5 days and then the average was calculated. For exercise average heart rate was measured continually during the 40 minutes of exercise for five days. At the end of each treatment period, each horse was individually led to a separate stable away from the other horses, thus placing them under mild social isolation conditions. This was a regular management practice for all the horse's on the yard as this was where each horse would be taken for shoeing, clipping, grooming and for routine veterinary treatment. The animal's behaviour was then monitored for 1 hour, with reactivity scores from 0 (no reaction) to 5 (extreme reaction) being taken every 2 minutes and then averaged (Momozawa *et al.*, 2003), Reactivity scores were analysed for significant differences using the Wilcoxons signed rank test. Heart rate was recorded at 5 s intervals using a Polar Heart Rate Monitor whilst each animal was observed. Average heart rates were calculated for each horse and these were then analysed, along with basal heart rates, using ANOVA.

Results

It was found that the reactivity scores for all horses were significantly higher when fed treatment S, than when the horses were fed treatment F ($P = 0.002$). Mean reactivity scores for each horse are presented in Table 1. The results indicate that experimental animals showed more stress-related behaviours when fed diet S, which can be seen by the higher mean reactivity scores.

Analysis of heart rate also found that heart rates were significantly ($P < 0.001$) higher when the horses were fed S, compared to when they were fed F, or compared to basal rates (Figure 1).

Table 1. Mean reactivity scores for horses fed a high starch, low fibre diet vs. a high fibre, low starch diet.

Diet	Mean reactivity score	s.e.d	P-value
High starch, low fibre	3	0.045	P=0.002
High fibre, low starch	1.1		

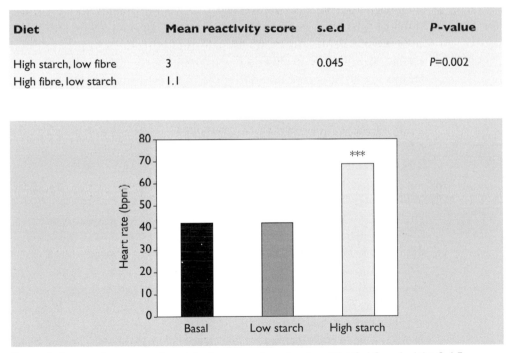

Figure 1. Average heart rate (bpm) for horses at base levels, whilst fed S and whilst fed F.
*** P<0.001; F stat 25.768

Discussion

Although few studies have been conducted to investigate the direct link between starch consumption and reactivity in horses, the current study appears to complement work that has alluded to such a link (Hothersall and Nicol, 2009). High starch diets are known to cause an increased glycaemic response, compared to diets high in fibre and/or fat (Treiber *et al.*, 2005) and consequently produce lowered behavioural reactivity (Nicol *et al.*, 2005; Holland *et al.*, 1996). Work carried out in rats subjected to microdialysis (Bequet *et al.*, 2001) found that increased levels of blood glucose corresponded with increased serotonin production in the hippocampus. Wurtman *et al.* (2003) found that increased levels of serotonin can produce increased reactivity, often manifested as increased performance of appetitive behaviours. Wurtman *et al.* (2003) found that an increased glycaemic peak initiated a heightened insulin response, which, in turn, diverted tyrosine from competitive places on carrier proteins destined to cross the blood:brain barrier, thus increasing the uptake of tryptophan into the brain. Serotonergic neurons found within the hippocampus respond to increases in tryptophan levels, resulting in increased serotonin production. Although this current study did not measure levels of plasma tryptophan:LNAA ratio (Large Neutral Amino Acids), it is postulated that the increased reactivity seen when the experimental horses consumed the high starch diets is a result of an increased glycaemic response and corresponding activation of serotonergic brain systems.

References

Béquet F, Gomez-Merino D, Berthelot M, Guezennec CY (2001) Exercise-induced changes in brain glucose and serotonin revealed by microdialysis in rat hippocampus: effect of glucose supplementation. Acta Physiologica Scandinavica 173:223-230.

Holland JL, Kronfeld DS, Meacham TN (1996) Behaviour of horses is affected by soy lecithin and corn oil in the diet. J Anim Sci 74:1252-1255.

Hothersall B and Nicol C (2009) Role of diet and feeding in normal and stereotypic behaviours in horses. Vet Clin Equine 25:167-181.

Nicol CJ, Badnell-Waters AJ, Bice R *et al.* (2005) The effects of diet and weaning method on the behaviour of young horses. Appl Anim Behav Sci 95:205-221.

NRC (2007) Nutritional Requirements of Horses. National Academies Press.

Ralston SL (2007) Evidence-based equine nutrition. Vet Clin North Am Equine Pract 23:365-384.

Treiber KH, Boston RC, Kronfeld DS *et al.* (2005) Insulin resistance and compensation in TB weanlings adapted to high-glycaemic meals. J Anim Sci 83:2357-2364.

Williams CA, Kronfeld DS, Staniar WB *et al.* (2001) Plasma glucose and insulin responses of TB mares fed a meal high in starch and sugar or fat and fibre. J Anim Sci 79:2196-2201.

Wurtman RJ, Wurtman JJ, Regan MM, McDermott JM, Tsay RH, Breu JJ (2003) Effects of normal meals rich in carbohydrates or proteins on plasma tryptophan and tyrosine ratios. Am J Clin Nutr 77:128–32.

Zeyner AC, Geißler C, Dittrich A (2004) Effects of hay intake and feeding sequence on variables in faeces and faecal water of horses. J Anim Physiol Anim Nutr 88:7-19.

A marine mineral supplement for Aquacid™

B.D. Nielsen[1], E.C. Ryan[2], C.I. O'Connor-Robison[1]

[1]Department of Animal Science, Michigan State University, 1287D Anthony Hall, East Lansing, MI, 48824-1225, USA; bdn@msu.edu

[2]Large Animal Clinical Sciences, Michigan State University, East Lansing, MI, 48824, USA

Take home message

The findings suggest that supplementation of a calcified seaweed supplement (Aquacid™) increased bone turnover of yearlings as compared with supplementation of limestone that provided an equivalent amount of calcium when fed with a diet containing the National Research Council recommended amount of calcium.

Introduction

A major issue faced by trainers of athletic horses is the prevention of skeletal injuries. Manipulation of diet and exercise are two management factors used to influence skeletal integrity. AquaCid™ (Marigot Ltd, Cork, Ireland) is a supplement produced from a calcified seaweed that is high in calcium and magnesium as well as other bone promoting minerals including silicon and boron. The objective of this study was to test whether supplementation of AquaCid™ can have a positive effect on the mineralization of the equine third metacarpus (MCIII) bone and markers of bone metabolism as compared with supplementation of limestone that provides an equivalent amount of calcium when fed with a diet containing the National Research Council (NRC) recommended amount of calcium.

Materials and methods

Fourteen yearlings were ranked according to radiographic bone aluminum equivalence (RBAE) and gender, were pair matched, and randomly assigned to two treatment groups. Each group was provided one of two mineral supplements in addition to their normal diet. The treated group (Aq) received 75 g AquaCid™/horse/day, which provided an additional 15 g of calcium. The control group (Co) received 39.5 g of limestone to provide a similar amount of calcium. The study lasted for 112 days, with blood being taken every 28 days. Additional radiographs were taken of the left third metacarpus of the 14 yearlings at day 56 and 112 to track changes in RBAE. RBAE of each cortex was calculated to estimate mineral content. Blood was analyzed for osteocalcin (a bone formation marker) and serum C-telopeptide crosslaps of type I collagen (a bone resorption marker) to detect alterations in bone metabolism.

Results and conclusions

Using day 0 values as a covariate for bone markers, there was a trend ($P = 0.07$) for osteocalcin concentrations to be greater in Aq horses than in Co. Likewise, C-telopeptide crosslaps of type I collagen concentrations were greater ($P < 0.0001$) in Aq horses than in Co. There were minimal differences in RBAE values.

In conclusion, supplementing AquaCid™ to young horses in an amount designed to provide calcium above NRC requirements produced altered bone metabolism compared with that in horses supplemented with limestone. These findings suggest AquaCid™, while not altering bone mass, increases bone turnover and may aid in repairing damaged bone and preventing injuries.

High level endurance training: descriptive study based on the follow-up of the French team over seasons 2009 and 2010

C. Robert[1], L. Mathews-Martin[2] and J.L. Leclerc[3]
[1]Ecole Nationale Vétérinaire d'Alfort, 94704 Maisons-Alfort cedex, France
[2]Domaine Barbette, 58300 Sougy sur Loire, France
[3]10 rue Christophe Doublat, 88000 Epinal, France

Take home message

A high-level endurance season is a succession of regular slow work and more intense work followed by recovery periods to minimize exercise induced troubles. Diet is based on forage and presents few variations during the season resulting in small changes in condition score.

Introduction

Endurance exercise is a high-demanding effort exposing horses to metabolic troubles and lameness. In all sports, prevention of exercise induced injuries is based on rational and adequate conditioning. However, very few information is available on endurance training in field conditions, most studies focusing either on responses to treadmill conditioning or endurance rides (Barton et al., 2003, Schott et al., 2006).

The purpose of the study was to get a picture of the management of elite endurance horses based on the follow-up of horses selected for the French national team for the European Championship in Assisi (2009) and the World Equestrian Games (WEG) in Lexington (2010).

Materials and methods

Horses and selection process

All horses selected as members of the French national team in 2009 and 2010 entered the study. At the beginning of the year, 15 riders were selected based on their performance the year before. They were asked to participate in a first training (T1) in March and a 160 km ride at the end of May (either Compiègne or Rambouillet). Following the 'selection rides', only horses placed in the 10 first remained in the selection while new horses entered the selection following their good performance in these rides. Horses were then examined in July (Training 2-T2), in August (T3) and just before their departure for the championship (T4). Final selection depended on the fitness of horses at T4 with 5 horses in the team for the European Championship and WEG.

Follow-up

At each training and at the selection ride, horses were assessed for fitness using body measurements (girth, skin fold), body condition score (BCS; scoring system of the French National Studs on a 5 grades scale modified with 0.25 grades), medical and locomotor examinations. Information on training regimen, feeding practices, and general horses' health were obtained from the riders using questionnaires. A field exercise test was performed at each training. It was adapted to the global fitness level of horses (Table 1). After the end of exercise, recovery was assessed using a heart-rate meter. Blood samples were collected with minimal restraint from a jugular vein into commercial evacuated tubes in the morning before morning meal while horses were in their box stall and 1 hour after the end of exercise.

Measured parameters and statistical analysis

Blood collected in EDTA coated tubes was used to assess haematology by flow cytometry on an ADVIA 120 Hematology System. Lithium heparin samples and serum tubes were centrifuged (10 min at 3000 g) and harvested plasma/serum was transferred to plastic tubes that remained at 4 °C until measurement of biochemical parameters on a RX Imola analyser. Rest and post-exercise blood values were compared using a Student's paired t test.

Table 1. Protocol for follow-up of horses selected in the national team during seasons 2009 and 2010.

Outcome	Training 1 T1	160 km ride	Training 2 T2	Training 3 T3	Training 4 T4
Period	March	End May	July	August	Mid-September
Exercise					
Length (km)	27+1.5+1.5	160	27+1.5+1.5	32+25+1.5+1.5	20
Speed (km/h)	20, 25, 27	18 to 20	20, 25, 27	20, 20, 25, 27	18
Blood tests					
Haematology, biochemistry, endocrinology	At rest + 1h after exercise	The day before the ride + 1 h after the ride	At rest + 1 h after exercise	At rest + 1 h after exercise	At rest
Lactates			End of exercise	End of exercise	
Horses (2009-2010)	16-15	11-12	11-11	9-8	5-5

The daily nutritional supplies were calculated from the INRA tables (Martin-Rosset, 1990).

Results

Horses and selection protocol

A total of 23 different riders entered national selection in 2009 and 2010 with 33 different horses: 22 Arabians, 4 Anglo-Arabians, 4 cross-Arabians and 3 Shagya (16 geldings, 17 mares). Mean age was 10.2 ± 2.0 years [8-16]. High level experience varied between 1 and 6 years, with qualifications varying from only 2 qualifications in CEI** (120 km) to 9 qualifications in CEI*** (160 km).

From the 16-15 horses present at T1 (number of horses in 2009 and 2010 respectively), 11-12 participated in the 160 km ride. After the ride, 8-3 horses from the initial selection were present at T2 and 3-8 new horses entered the selection. Most horses present at T2 were present at T3. Reasons for withdrawal were a disappointing result at selection ride (32%), lameness either at training or during the ride

(48%), injury (1 horse), colic (1 horse), sale (2 horses) and size of the final team (2 horses). From final selection, 2 horses finished (3rd and 4th place) and 3 were eliminated for lameness at the EuCh; all horses finished the ride (4th, 8th, 10th, 11th and 33rd place) at the WEG.

Training and feeding practices

During winter, all except the young horses were on pasture 8 to 24 hours/day with no training at all. Training usually began in February depending on weather conditions. Between March and September, all horses had daily access to paddocks. Basal activity consisted in outdoor rides at walk for a mean duration of 2 hours, every two days or 3 days a week. For half of the horses, training also included sessions at trot and canter especially for horses trained in flat regions (from 10 minutes to one hour depending on the horse, the terrain and fitness level). In the final preparation phase, before the rides and T3, specific training sessions at canter were performed by all riders every 10 days on average (mean of 1:07 h, range 0:45-1:30).

After the 160 km ride, horses were given one month recovery (21-45 days).

Feeding practices were consistent with recommendations for elite endurance horses (Harris, 2009). For all horses, the basic diet consisted of good quality meadow hay regardless of the intensity of work. All horses except one were fed commercial feeds; 13 horses were also fed barley. Forage intake was impossible to estimate accurately. For the 18 horses fed hay *ad libitum*, this quantity was calculated from the total dry matter intake of horses in moderate to high level of training (2.5% BW, Martin-Rosset 1990). Forage usually represented more than 75% [52-93%] of total dry matter intake and supplied up to the 2/3 of the daily energy requirements (Table 2). During high level training periods, horses tended to receive a little less forage and more concentrates, even though, the total amount of energy per day did not vary significantly (mean 6.7 UFC). Only 2 of the 23 riders used vegetable oil to increase the energy amount of the diet during high intensity training periods. As a consequence, dry matter intake, fat percentage of the concentrates, total protein supply and MADc/UFC ratio did not change significantly all along the training season (Table 2). Twelve horses received mineral and vitamin supplements and 17

Table 2. Mean daily feed supply in 30 elite endurance horses; mean [min-max] values depending on the level of training.

	Training intensity	Low-to-moderate (T1 and T2)		High (ride and T3)	
Forage	Quantity (kg)	8.5	[5-11]	7.9	[5-12]
	Energy (UFC)	4.6	[2.7-6]	4.3	[2.7-6.5]
Concentrate	Quantity (kg)	2.2	[0.8-5.6]	2.5	[0.8-4.6]
	Energy (UFC)	2	[0.7-4.5]	2.3	[0.9-4.7]
Total	DM (kg)	9.6	[6.0-12.7]	9.4	[6.5-11.9]
	DM (kg/100 kg BW)	2.2	[1.4-2.9]	2.3	[1.6-2.8]
	% forage/total	79	[52-93]	75	[52-92]
	Fat (%)	6	[2-14]	5	[2-11]
	Energy (UFC)	6.7	[5.3-8.9]	6.7	[5.0-8.3]
	MADc (g)	697	[460-962]	693	[482-962]
	MADc/UFC	103	[90-112]	103	[91-116]

UFc = Unité Fourragère cheval ; MADc = Matière Azotée Digestible cheval; BW = Body weight in kg.

horses nutritional supplements (for muscles, joints, hoof ...). Only 4 horses were regularly supplemented with electrolytes and 4 others were offered electrolytes during the rides only.

After the training tests and the compétition horses were walked for 10 to 15 minutes, given a shower then rested in a box with hay. They were usually fed concentrates twice a day, i.e. in the morning and the evening.

Fitness evaluation and exercise tests

Riders voluntarily maintained horses over their optimal weight during low level training periods (T1 and T2) to achieve optimal weight during final intense preparation before the rides. However, body condition score did not show significant variations during the season (min 2.96 ± 0.24 at T3 and max 3.17 ± 0.38 at T1).

All horses completed the exercise tests without any difficulty. At T1 and T2, respectively 12.5 and 17.6% of the horses had a recovery time

(= time for HR≤64 bpm) higher than 10 minutes. Mean recovery time after each loop at T3 test was 1 min 34 sec [39 sec-6 min].

Blood analysis

Blood samples taken at rest showed consistent changes associated with endurance training (McGowan, 2008; McKeever, 1987; Muñoz *et al.*, 2002; Robert *et al.*, 2010), even at the beginning of the season: urea, total protein and alkaline phosphatase concentration was higher than the reference values in 100, 75 and 66% of the horses respectively. Training was associated with an increase in creatine kinase and sodium concentrations and a decrease in chloremia ($P < 0.05$).

After exercise, horses always presented some leucocytosis and neutrophilia, which is a normal finding (Barton *et al.*, 2003; Schott *et al.*, 2006). Signs of dehydration were significant after the ride and T3 only. Increases in total bilirubin, creatine kinase and serum amyloid A concentrations appeared proportional with the intensity of exercise (T2 < T3 < ride).

Conclusions

To our knowledge, this is the first study describing maintenance, training and fitness evaluation in elite endurance horses. Lameness appears to be the main reason for failure during the season. The results presented here can serve as training guidance for riders and trainers preparing horses for 120 to 160 km endurance rides.

Acknowledgements

This work was funded by the French Horse and Riding Institution *(IFCE)* and the French Ministry of Agriculture.

References

Barton MH, Williamson L, Jacks S, Norton N (2003) Body weight, hematological findings, and serum and plasma biochemical findings of horses competing in a 48-, 83-, or 159-km endurance ride under similar terrain and weather conditions. Am J vet Res 64:746-753.

Harris P (2009) Feeding management of elite endurance horses. Vet Clin North Am Equine Pract 25:137-53.

Martin-Rosset W (1990) Alimentation des chevaux. Ed. INRA Editions, Versailles pp. 232.

McGowan C (2008) Clinical pathology in the racing horse: the role of clinical pathology in assessing fitness and performance in the racehorse. Vet Clin North Am Equine Pract 24: 405-421.

McKeever KH, Schurg WA, Jarrett SH, Convertino VA (1987) Exercise training-induced hypervolemia in the horse. Med Sci Sports Exerc 19:21-27.

Muñoz A, Riber C, Santisteban R, Lucas RG, Castejón FM (2002) Effect of training duration and exercise on blood-borne substrates, plasma lactate and enzyme concentrations in Andalusian, Anglo-Arabian and Arabian breeds. Eq vet J Suppl 34:245-251.

Robert C, Goachet A-G, Mathews-Martin L, Grezy L, Fraipont A, Votion D, Van Erck E, Leclerc J-L (2010) Hydration and electrolyte balance in horses during an endurance season. Eq Vet J Suppl: 38:98-104.

Schott H, Marlin DJ, Geor RJ, Holbrook TC, Deaton CM, Vincent T, Dacre K, Schroter, RC, Cunilleras JE, Cornelisse CJ (2006) Changes in selected physiological and laboratory measurements in elite horses competing in a 160 km endurance ride. Eq Vet J 36:37-42.

Workload during an eventing competition

E. Valle[1,3], R. Odore[2], P. Badino[2], E. Fraccaro[2], C. Girardi[2], R. Zanatta[2] and B. Bergero[1,3]

[1]Department of Animal Production, Epidemiology and Ecology, Faculty of Veterinary Medicine, Italy; emanuela.valle@unito.it
[2]Department of animal pathology Faculty of Veterinary Medicine, University of Torino, Italy
[3]International Centre of the Horse, Druento, Italy

Take home message

Information on workload during eventing competition is provided. The training methods of horses should be based on exercises and skills required, but also on heart rate (HR) that horses reach and maintain during the competition.

Introduction

Eventing is recognized as one of the most demanding equestrian disciplines (Murray et al., 2006); participants are involved in different tests: dressage, judged on the quality of gaits, and precision of movements (Williams et al., 2009), jumping, where ability skills are verified and cross-country, where strength and boldness of both horse and rider are tested (Marlin, 2007). Today most of the competitions are organized in the so-called short form (SF), introduced for the first time in 2004 in prestigious competitions such as the Rolex Kentucky CCI 4 (Murray et al., 2006).

Monitoring horses during competition can help to focus the training regimes that elicit adaptations appropriate for the sport being participated in (Williams et al., 2009). Measurement of heart rate (HR) during exercise has been shown to be an objective tool for estimating the workload of horses and monitoring responses to training. The majority of research on HR responses to exercise were conducted during standardized exercise tests on high-speed treadmills (Dekker et al., 2007).

To the authors knowledge there is not much literature on the description of the effort required by horses to complete a SF event, both for elite horses (advanced level; AL) or general purpose horses (intermediate level; IL).

The present study was undertaken to get information on the workload of IL and AL horses during an eventing competition using HR as index. Moreover the duration and the intensity of warm-up (WU), and relationships between HR and speed (S) as well as HR recovery (HRR) after the cross country phase were evaluated.

Materials and methods

Competition features

Data were collected during an official two days event in Cameri Sport Club in the north of Italy in May 2009. The weather condition remained relatively constant through the two days of competition (mean temperature 19 °C, relative humidity 66%). In the first day horses performed the dressage (Dr) and show jumping (Sj) tests. On the second day the horses performed the cross-country (Cr). All the tests were between 8:30 - 11:30 a.m. and the grass ground condition, was similar for all horses, irrespective of starting order. The description of the competition features is reported in Table 1.

Table 1. Description of the competition features.

Level	Dressage test	Show-jumping test	Cross-country test
Intermediate level	E206 [a]	Distance 390 m	Distance 2460 m
		Speed 350 m/min	Speed 510 m/min
		Time 67 s	Time 4:50 min
		Fence height 1.10 m	Fence height 1.05 m
Advanced level	E310/F200 [b]	Distance 400 m	Distance 2700 -3100 m
		Speed 350 /min	Speed 520-530 m/min
		Time 69 s	Time 5:20-5:51 min
		Fence height 1.15/1.20 m	Fence height 1.10-1.15 m

[a] Marks were given for medium walk, working-medium-trot and working canter.

[b] Marks were given for medium-extended walk, working-medium-collected trot, working-medium-collected canter and shoulder in at trot and rein back.

Animals

10 warmblood horses (7 geldings, one stallion and 2 mares; 5 AL, 5 IL) were recruited (Table 2). All horses were kept in the same stable and trained by the same trainer. Horses regularly participated in competitions.

Data collection

Horses were equipped with a HR monitor and GPS system (Polar Equine RS800 G3™). The belt with electrodes was placed under the saddle before the horses left the box for the WU and competition phase (C). The recording watch was set to record every 5 s. The GPS was applied directly to the saddle to maximize reception of the satellites. Veterinary students were assigned to each horse to identify the horse during the trial and record the time of start and finish respectively for WU or C phase for each test (Dr, Sj, Cr). Horses were tested two weeks before the competition on track in an exercise session to obtain their maximum HR (Table 2). Running distance was 1,250 m and riders were asked to run their horses at maximal speed. To encourage the riders to exercise their horses sufficiently they were told the calculated HRmax that their horses should be able to achieve by substracting the age of the horses from 230 bpm.

Data manipulation

HR and GPS data were evaluated with Polar Pro trainer 5™ equine edition software to identify: mean HR (%HRMean), maximum HR (%HRMax), speed (S, m/min), duration (D, min) respectively for WU or C in each test. For Cr data of HRR in the first 3 minutes after the end of competition were used. To compare the workload of horses, all HR data were expressed as percentage of maximum HRmax.

Table 2. Age of horses and highest HR (bpm) during a fast gallop exercise session (HRfast).

	Age, years (min-max)	Highest HR recorded, (Range, bpm)
Advanced level	9-13	200-213
Intermediate level	6-13	190-228

Table 3. Mean heart rate (HR), maximum heart rate expressed as % of the HRfast (maximum HR recorded during a fast exercise session), during warm-up and competition between advanced and intermediate level horses for each test.

	Test[1]	Category	Mean	SD	P
Warm up	%DrHRMax	Intermediate	68.6	±10.8	0.05
		Advanced	58.0	± 5.92	
	%DrHRMean	Intermediate	45.4	± 2.51	0.04
		Advanced	42.2	± 2.59	
	%SjHRMax	Intermediate	77.6	± 7.16	0.36
		Advanced	79.2	± 5.93	
	%SjHRMean	Intermediate	51.2	± 6.30	0.05
		Advanced	45.6	± 2.41	
	%CrHRMax	Intermediate	83.0	± 3.94	0.13
		Advanced	80.6	± 2.19	
	%CrHRMean	Intermediate	52.6	± 3.85	0.21
		Advanced	54.2	± 1.79	
Competition	%DrHRmax	Intermediate	65.8	± 2.77	<0.01
		Advanced	57.2	± 3.63	
	%DrHRMean	Intermediate	54.4	± 4.34	0.01
		Advanced	48.2	± 1.92	
	%SjHRMax	Intermediate	88.6	± 8.20	0.38
		Advanced	89.8	± 1.48	
	% SjHRMean	Intermediate	73.0	± 6.04	0.12
		Advanced	76.6	± 2.07	
	%CrHRMax	Intermediate	96.2	± 3.90	0.09
		Advanced	99.0	± 1.00	
	%CrHRMean	Intermediate	83.4	±11.3	0.06
		Advanced	93.6	± 2.30	

[1] %HRMean: mean heart rate; %HRMax: maximum heart rate; Dr: Dressage; Sj: Show jumping; Cr: Cross Country.

Statistical analysis

All the data were analysed using SPSS 17.0® software. The level of significance was set at $P < 0.05$. For each test (Dr, Sj, Cr) data were analyzed by one tailed unpaired t-test to check in which group (AL or IL) HRMean, %HRMax, speed (m/min), duration (min) during WU or

C would be higher. The relationships between HR and S for WU and C phase were determined using one tailed Person's correlations. The relationship between HR decrease and recovery time was investigated by multiple nonlinear curve estimation procedures using data from seven horses (4 AL, 3 IL). The model with the highest coefficient of determination (r^2) was accepted as the optimal model for the relationship.

Results

Differences during WU and C between AL and IL are reported in Table 3. During Dr, IL horses had higher %HRMean and %HRMax during WU and C. During Sj differences were recorded only for WU with higher values for IL horses. No significant differences between horse groups were observed for WU before Cr, but %HRMean was tendentially higher in AL than in IL horses during the C phase.

No differences were recorded in the distance worked during the WU before all competition phases. No differences were recorded in the duration of WU for Dr and Cr between AL and IL, but AL spent more time for WU during Sj. No differences were identified for maximum speed, but during the WU of Sj IL horses had higher mean speeds (Table 4).

Table 4. Duration, distance worked, mean and maximum speed during warm-up between advanced and intermediate level horses for each test.

Warm-up	Category	Dressage			Show jumping			Cross country		
		Mean	SD	P	Mean	SD	P	Mean	SD	P
Duration	Intermediate	39.6	±19.9	0.34	16.4	± 8.99	0.04	28.4	± 7.80	0.46
(min)	Advanced	35.0	±13.0		31.8	±13.5		28.0	± 2.55	
Distance	Intermediate	4.14	± 2.05	0.45	2.15	± 0.95	0.11	11.0	± 15.7	0.20
(km)	Advanced	4.28	± 1.51		3.55	± 1.83		4.40	± 0.43	
Mean speed	Intermediate	134	±18.8	0.50	170	±32.6	0.05	119	± 63.5	0.07
(m/min)	Advanced	134	±18.8		137	± 9.00		170	± 10.0	
Max speed	Intermediate	258	±35.5	0.35	380	±70.0	0.10	379	±117	0.19
(m/min)	Advanced	248	±41.7		321	±38.1		433	± 43.4	

No correlations were identified between speed and HR during the WU or C for Dr. No correlations were identified for WU before Cr, while for C there was one ($P=0.004$; $r=0.78$); no correlations were identified for WU before Sj, but for C this was the case ($P=0.05$; $r=-0.60$).

The mean percentage of HRfast at the end of the competition was $91.6\pm9.72\%$. After 180 seconds it was 52.7 ± 7.88. The power curve appeared to describe the phenomenon in the proper way ($r^2=0.92$).

For the AL group the maximal calculated HR (230 minus age) was 219 ± 2 bpm while the maximal HR measured during the fast gallop on the 1,250 m track was 206 ± 5. The difference between the theoretical and the recorded HR max was 13 bpm. For the IL group of horses the respective values were 221 ± 3 bpm, 208 ± 14 bpm and 13 bpm.

Discussion

Dressage

The duration of WU was similar to that observed in another study conducted on dressage horses (Williams *et al.*, 2009). The %HRMax and %HRMean during WU were higher for IL horses. This could be due to the different levels of preparation of horses and riders of this group. Under 150-160 bpm (Williams *et al.*, 2009) HR could be influenced by excitement and stress and not just by effort. This is also confirmed by the lack of correlation between S and HR rate for this phase of the competition.

Show jumping

The WU phase was longer in the AL group (32 vs 16 min) in agreement with the study on Sj horses of Whitaker *et al.* (2008); horses of the higher competitive level were warmed up more. The %mean HR during WU was higher for IL horses, but this could be due to the higher speed reached during this phase of competition. The negative correlation between S and HR during the C phase could be related to the fact that HR may be influenced by other factors than exercise effort such as excitation.

Cross country

The WU duration was similar for both horse groups (28 minutes); there were no obvious differences in HR during the WU or C but for just a tendency for AL horses to have higher %MeanHR during C. The relationship between the HR and speed was stronger during this phase of the competition. The HRR recovery showed a decrease to 53% of the HRfast 180 seconds after competition (Figure 1). Similar findings were described by Bitschnau *et al.* (2010) in warmblood horses during a treadmill test.

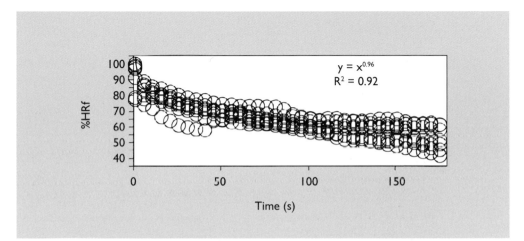

Figure 1. Percentage of post exercise heart rate recovery (HRR). Raw data (dots) and mean regression line.

Conclusions

Training methods should be based on exercises and skills required of horses, but also on the HR that horses reach and maintain during competition. To analyse the different workloads in terms of % of maximum HR it is necessary to provide objective data to the riders.

References

Bitschnau C, Wiestner T, Trachsel DS, Auer JA, Weishaupt MA (2010) Performance parameters and post exercise heart rate recovery in Warmblood sports horses of different performance levels. Equine vet J 42:17-22.

Dekker H, Marlin D, Alexander L, Bishop R, Harris P (2007) A pilot study investigating the relationship between perceived and actual workload and estimated energy intake in riding centre horses. Comp Exerc Physiol 4:7-14.

Marlin DJ (2007) Exercise Physiology of Eventing. www.davidmarlin.co.uk.

Murray JK, Senior JM, Singer ER (2006) A comparison of cross-country recovery rates at CCI 2* with and without steeplechase competitions. Equine Vet J Suppl 36:133-138.

Williams RJ, Chandlera RE, Marlin DJ (2009) Heart rates of horses during competitive dressage. Comp Exerc Physiol 6:7-15.